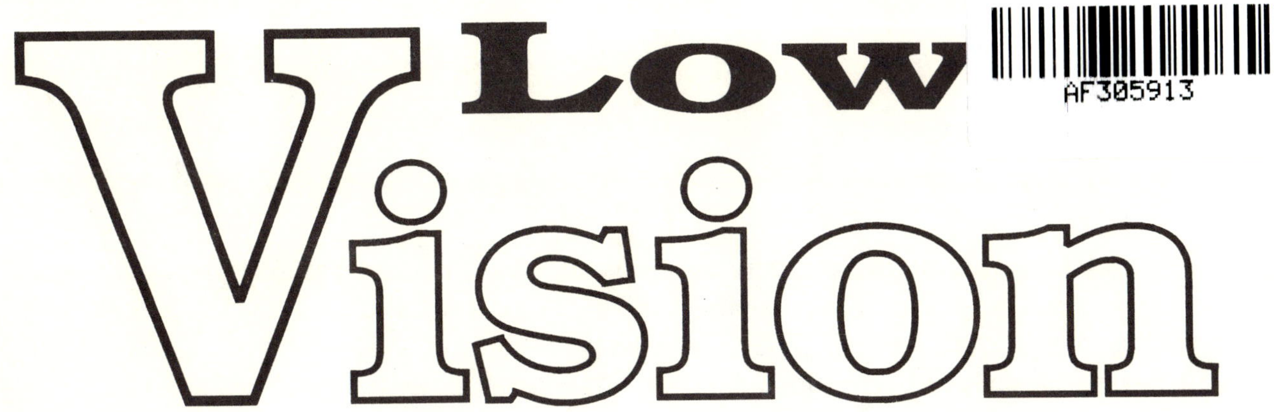

Low Vision

A Resource Guide with Adaptations for Students with Visual Impairments

by

Nancy Levack

with contributions from
Gretchen Stone
and
Virginia Bishop

Design and Layout by
Brigitte MaGee

Texas School for the Blind and Visually Impaired

Printed in the United States of America.

First Printing, December 1991.

Copies of this publication may be ordered from:
Texas School for the Blind and Visually Impaired
Business Office
1100 West 45th Street
Austin, Texas 78756-3494

Library of Congress Cataloging-in-Publication Data
Levack, Nancy, 1944-
    Low vision : A resource guide with adaptations for students with visual impairments / by Nancy Levack ; with contributions from Gretchen Stone and Virginia Bishop.
    p. 280
    Includes bibliographical references and index.
    ISBN 1-880366-04-5 : $10.00
    1. Visually handicapped children--Education--Handbooks, manuals, etc. 2. Vision disorders in children--Handbooks, manuals, etc. 3. Visually handicapped children--Education--United States--Handbooks, manuals, etc. I. Stone, Gretchen. II. Bishop, Virginia E. III. Title.
    HV1626.L48 1991
    371.91'1--dc20   91-40055
                                              CIP

Photographs: Bill Liles, TSBVI, Austin, TX
Illustrations: Brigitte MaGee, TSBVI, Austin, TX
Printing: AlphaGraphics, Austin, TX

Contents

Purpose of the Resource Guide

Chapter I

Components of Programming

Chapter II

Psychosocial Implications of Visual Impairment   *Chapter VIII*

Appendices

When Nancy Levack, the contributors, and advisors undertook a project to compile, in one volume, a comprehensive guide to low vision for the professional or parent of the 1990's, the task seemed exceedingly ambitious. The guide would reflect current philosophies, provide up-to-date medical, optical, and technical information, and include methodologies and adaptations which are practical while not intended to be a "here's how you do it" manual. This guide, *Low Vision: A Resource Guide with Adaptations for Students with Visual Impairments,* includes all of these characteristics and, in 1990's terminology, they have succeeded in making it, "user friendly"!

This guide is a compendium of resources and recommended adaptations. This guide contains information on functional vision assessments, media assessments, and assessments for distinguishing between learning and visual disabilities. This guide contains information on commonly encountered medical conditions, their treatments, and their educational implications. This guide includes optical and nonoptical approaches to provide a "least restrictive access to the visual environment" for students with low vision. This guide includes information on computer access and information on other electronic approaches to solve the challenges of low vision. This guide discusses how students with multiple physical and/or mental impairments and who have low vision may enhance their use of vision while the professional is asked to consider instructional priorities. And, this guide offers clear and forthright insight into the psychological implications of living with low vision.

The reader will find the recommended forms, lists of readings, tables, diagrams, and photographs most helpful in utilizing the guide. The author and contributors have the combined experience of teaching, writing, occupational therapy, and professional preparation. They called upon these experiences as they carefully chose the best ways in which to present their information.

As a teacher-educator in the 1990's, and as someone with personal low vision experiences, I enthusiastically welcome this new guide to the professional literature. A great many students with low vision will undoubtedly benefit from this publication.

Anne L. Corn, Ed. D.
Professor and Coordinator,
Programs for the Visually Handicapped
The University of Texas at Austin

When the decision was made to write a sensory perception curriculum, Robin Loumiet, the curriculum director at the time, and I agonized about whether it was appropriate to develop a list of skills with corresponding methods and materials, as was the plan for the rest of the curriculum. Our biggest concern was that we did not want to imply that programming in the use of the senses was a separate curricular area like social studies or math. We felt that instruction in the use of the senses must be infused into all other curricular areas. As I began to research the issue, I found that the abundance of information and complexity of the issues involved in the use of vision merited producing a guide that focused exclusively on low vision.

Once the decision was made to concentrate on vision, it became clear to me that I would have the opportunity to offer teachers and parents a synthesis as well as a guide to this large body of material. The goal of this project, therefore, has been the creation of a book which included everything that I wished I had at my fingertips when I was programming for students in my classroom.

The task seemed overwhelming. I remembered the days as a classroom teacher when I poured over a student's file trying to get clues about how and what she could see. I remember the panic I felt when I tried to do a functional vision assessment and secretly worried, "Am I really seeing what I think I see?". And I remember the confusion and frustration that I felt when I finally had an assessment down on paper and still wasn't sure what kind of lessons might be helpful to the student.

On the basis of those memories, I tried to include in the guide what would have been helpful to me in meeting those challenges. I then asked teachers who were currently working with students with visual impairments to give me feedback and suggestions. It wasn't long before I realized that what we had was "low vision stone soup". Just as in the fable, I made the pebble broth; but as people read, commented on and added to the drafts, the soup acquired its rich seasoning and additional ingredients.

I have no illusion that one book will answer the challenges related to programming for students who have low vision. Practice and experience working with students is the *real* source of information.

There are some people who must be singled out for recognition in this project. Robin Loumiet asked me to do the project in the first place and then sat across the room radiating confidence that there really would be a guide when I had my deepest doubts. Brigitte MaGee was the person with whom I worked most closely on this project. She created a layout for my words that made them look credible, even before I believed them. While I created most of the words, Brigitte created the *book*.

I will always be grateful to Gretchen Stone, who took time away from preparation for the defense of her doctoral dissertation and her other full time jobs to write the chapter Physical Conditions, the Sensory Systems, and How They Affect Visual Performance. Ginny Bishop was involved in the beginning and the end of the project. She wrote some sections on sensory perception for an earlier curriculum project which we borrowed for this guide, and then reviewed the draft with a fine tooth comb and rewrote some of the information in the chapter on Medical Information Related to Visual Impairment. Anne Corn has reviewed the entire manuscript at a few junctures and provided valuable suggestions and challenges.

Then there are all of the people who are listed on page xii. Vivian Caldwell, Lynne Lampert and Robin Loumiet contributed sections for specific topics within the chapters. The advisors and consultants reviewed the entire manuscript, gave helpful information, and offered editorial suggestions. Some consultants used the guide with their students and offered valuable feedback. Phil Hatlen and Cyral Miller provided administrative and personal support.

Finally, I am particularly grateful to my friend, Millie Smith, who taught the first course I ever took about low vision, and who, during my teaching years, was only a few classrooms away and always helpful whenever I had pithy questions like "What does this student see and what do I do about it?". When Millie said that she liked the guide, I felt that I had done what I had set out to do.

Nancy Levack, December 1991

Acknowledgements

Other Contributors	Advisors	Consultants
Vivian Caldwell	Natalie Barraga	Nan Bulla
Lynn Lampert	Anne Corn	Sylvia Carnes
Robin Loumiet	Randall Jose	Lila Coughran
	Nancy Patton	Bill Daugherty
	Sharon Zell Sacks	Linda Donovan
	Rosanne Silberman	Jim Durkel
		Miles Fain
		Kathy Geiger
		Kitra Hill
		Susan Hauser
		Pamala King
		Bill Koehler
		Stephanie Labossiere
		Fran LaWare
		Linda Locke
		Fred Martinez
		Ken Miller
		Ann Moore
		Ouida Fae Morris
		Pat Muller
		Lauren Newton
		Susan Osterhaus
		Susan Otey
		Brenda O'Sail
		Carol Ramberg
		Eileen Reed
		Stacy Shafer
		Renae Shepler
		Mildred Smith
		Chris Strickling
		Frankie Swift
		Sharon Trusty
		Garner Vogt
		Mary Wikoff
		Faye White

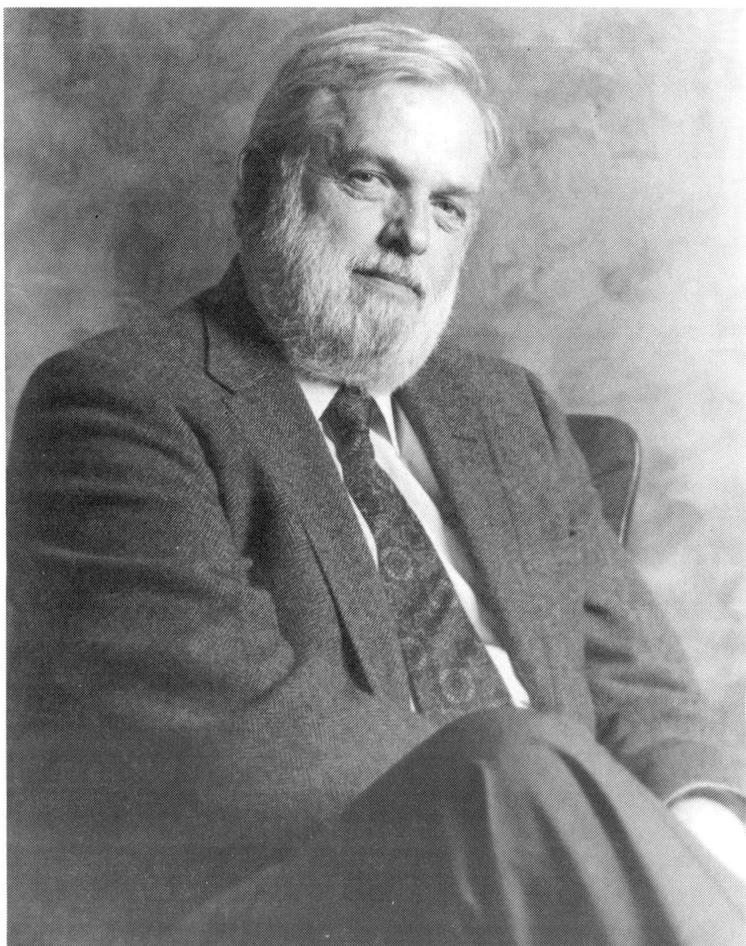

The photograph of Phil Hatlen was done by a junior photography student at TSBVI as part of a unit in studio portraiture. Cassie White is a low vision student in her third semester of photography under instructor Carrell Grigsby. Cassie helped paint the backdrop, set up the studio lights, metered the subject from all sides, and calculated exposures for manual settings on an autofocus 35mm camera. She was independent in the film and print processing to produce this perfect print.

Phil Hatlen, Superintendent, 1990-
Texas School for the Blind and Visually Impaired
Austin, Texas

This photo is an illustration of a skill which can be taught to, and enjoyed by, persons with low vision. It may come as a surprise to some that TSBVI offers photography classes to visually impaired students. This is just one example of how innovations in low vision utilization can expand the opportunities, learning, and enjoyment of visually impaired persons.

It is fitting that this publication is written by a member of the faculty of TSBVI, and that it is available for purchase through TSBVI. This guide exists because of the pioneering work of Dr. Natalie Barraga, Professor Emeritus, University of Texas, and once a teacher at TSBVI. Dr. Barraga's dramatic findings in 1963 regarding the effects of low vision utilization and low vision stimulation began a profound redirection in how students with low vision would learn. We acknowledge with deep appreciation the work of Dr. Barraga, our neighbor, and we hope you will find this publication useful as we continue to implement and expand Dr. Barraga's findings.

Philip H. Hatlen, Ed.D.

Purpose
of the
Resource Guide

The major purposes of this guide are:

• To provide guidelines for assessing students' visual functioning

• To provide guidelines for planning and implementing programming that will enhance students' visual functioning

• To serve as a reference guide for information related to low vision

In order to keep this document a manageable size, this information is usually limited in detail. However, whenever possible books and articles of particular merit have been included at the end of each chapter under the heading "Additional Readings and Resources". When specific sections of a book apply, this has been noted. It is hoped that these references will give the instructor information about where to go for additional or more detailed information when needed.

This guide has been written for people who are responsible for educational programming for students who are visually impaired. These include teachers who are certified to teach students who are visually impaired, teachers who are certified to teach students who have dual-sensory impairments, and orientation and mobility instructors. Other people who might find this information useful include parents and others in regular and special education who work with students who are visually impaired, including teachers, related services staff, and administrators.

Intended Users

This guide is intended for use with students who are eligible for educational services based on the unique educational needs created by their visual impairment. Because programming can begin at birth, this document pertains to students who are any age from birth through twenty-one years of age. In this document, visual impairment refers to identified organic differences in the visual system which are so severe that even after medical and conventional optical intervention, the student is unable to receive an appropriate education within the regular educational setting without special education services designed for those who are visually impaired.

Intended Student Population

If students have been diagnosed as having no or immeasurable visual acuity, the instructor will need to review the records carefully for the cause of the blindness and observe the student carefully to determine if the student might have some functional vision. A functional vision assessment should be done. If it is determined that the student has no functional vision, there may be some general information on anatomy and eye conditions in this guide that might be helpful, but this guide will provide little information for programming.

Components
of Programming

Philosophy

Several concepts have influenced decisions about the content of this guide and can also guide decisions about appropriate programming for students. These include:

- Every student has **unique needs and differences** which must be assessed and respected when planning a program of instruction in the use of low vision.

- **Skills in the use of vision should be infused in all the areas of the students' day,** not taught in isolation as a separate instructional topic.

- **Students must be involved in the decision-making process** to the best of their abilities. This includes respecting and using what is motivating to them, listening to them when they identify the visual skills that they need and/or wish to acquire, and observing them carefully, particularly if they are nonverbal, in order to determine what they need.

- **All decisions** about programming should be **based on** whether a particular intervention fosters **further independence.**

- **A transdisciplinary approach should be used** in determining
  individual program needs and carrying out recommendations. The
  student, parent, other agency representatives, and medical, instructional, and support staff should work together as members of the
  team in a cooperative effort to design and carry out programming.

- Effective programming should be based on identifying the challenges that a student's visual impairment imposes and, whenever
  possible, suggesting intervention that allows the student to function
  in the **least restrictive visual environment,** this means as little
  adaptation as needed to function effectively.

- An understanding of the developmental sequence of visual abilities
  often helps an instructor to know if a specific objective is reasonable
  for a student. However, some students may not follow the "developmental sequence" in their acquisition of efficient use of their low
  vision. Consequently while information about the developmental
  sequence of visual abilities is included, **this guide focuses mainly
  on the immediate functional needs of the student.**

- Effective programming for students who are visually impaired should
  include a **clinical low vision evaluation.** This information is vital to
  the optimum planning for any student with visual impairments and for
  selecting the best learning medium.

The Challenge of Programming for Students Who Are Visually Impaired

The primary purpose of programming for students who have low vision is to "overcome the handicapping effects of their visual (or sight) impairment, function at an optimal level, and live a comfortable life-style" (Jose, 1983, p. 62). There are many challenges to the implementation of this ambitious goal.

- **Students who are visually impaired comprise a diverse population** in terms of ages, cognitive abilities, and types of eye conditions. The seriousness of the condition can range from mild to profound. When programming, there are no easy answers that generalize to all students with visual impairments. The instructor must be knowledgeable about all of these factors and then take them into consideration when recommending a program which attempts to meet the student's individual needs.

- **Successful programming often depends on the commitment and consistency maintained by all the members of the interdisciplinary team** including the students, the students' family, and other educational and medical professionals who work with the students. It is sometimes difficult to get this level of consistency among such a diverse group. The instructor must work to get this consistency and to get consensus about what are the priorities that will be worked on as goals and objectives.

- **The field is constantly changing and the instructor must keep informed** on current research and technology, as well as current practices in the education of students with severe and multiple disabilities.

- **The instructor must be able to establish and maintain rapport with students and their families** and to assist them, as well as other educational staff members, in developing realistic expectations for the students.

- **The instructor must have knowledge of the variety of service delivery systems** available to students who are visually impaired.

A thorough discussion of the role and responsibilities of instructors who are certified to work with students who are visually impaired can be found in *Program Planning and Evaluation for Blind and Visually Impaired Students: National Guidelines for Educational Excellence* (Hazekamp & Huebner, 1989, pp. 25-27, 71-74). These responsibilities can be extensive and may vary depending on the needs of the individual student. A brief synopsis of the role of the instructor would include responsibilities in the areas of assessment, educational programming, and providing support for students, parents, regular education personnel and sighted peers. Specific responsibilities include:

ASSESSMENT

- Do functional vision assessments with input from the students and whenever possible, the students' family, and significant school staff.

- Determine the most efficient learning media for each student, as well as the most efficient literary media, when appropriate.

- Assist in other assessments (e. g., psychological).

- Recommend other related assessments (e. g., occupational therapy, physical therapy, speech and language, auditory, learning disabilities).

- Recommend further low vision consultations to determine if any medical interventions would improve the students' visual functioning or restore any possible vision.

EDUCATIONAL PROGRAMMING

- Provide specialized instruction related to the students' unique needs as persons who have a visual impairment, particularly in the following areas:
    - sensory perception
    - basic cognitive abilities
    - psycho-social development
    - knowledge of visual impairment and self-advocacy
    - verbal and nonverbal communication
    - learning and literacy media, and adaptations for reading, writing, and use of computers
    - adaptations for other academic subjects
    - physical abilities
    - orientation and mobility
    - self-care
    - recreation
    - adaptations for sexuality education
    - career awareness, employability skills, and transition.
    (Educating Students with Visual Impairments, 1991, p. 5)

- Coordinate the instruction in skills related to the student's visual impairment with the students' parents, classroom teachers, related service staff and other professionals in the field of education of students who are visually impaired.

- Suggest environmental adjustments and adaptations which will improve the students' visual efficiency, and teach students to use them effectively when necessary.

- Obtain supplementary materials, educational aids and equipment that will be needed by the students.

- Provide support for **students** in the following ways:
    - understand their needs, their eye conditions and the implications
      for visual functioning
    - help students to understand their own attitudes and the attitudes
      of others related to their visual impairment
    - identify resources, services and support that are available lo-
      cally, from the state, and nationally
    - help students to develop realistic understanding of their abilities,
      progress, and future goals.

- Provide support for **parents** in the following ways:
    - help parents to understand the needs of their child, his eye
      condition and the implications for visual functioning
    - understand the parents' attitudes and the attitudes of others
      related to their child's visual impairment
    - identify resources, services and support that are available lo-
      cally, from the state, and nationally
    - help parents to develop realistic understanding of their child's
      abilities, progress, and future goals.

- Provide support for **regular education personnel** in the following ways:
    - help them to understand the needs of the students, including
      their eye condition and the implications for visual functioning
    - help them to understand their own attitudes and the attitudes of
      others related to visual impairment
    - identify resources, services and support that are available lo-
      cally, from the state, and nationally
    - help them to develop realistic understanding of their student's
      abilities, progress, and future goals.

- Provide support for the students' **sighted peers** in the following ways:
  - help them to understand their own attitudes and the attitudes of others related to visual impairment
  - help them to understand ways that they can support their class-mates who are visually impaired.

- Provide support for the **student in the community** in the following ways:
  - provide information about the importance of integrating disabled people in the community
  - provide help in developing adaptations which can support indi-viduals with disabilities in their work in the community
  - explore ways to provide employment and social opportunities within the community.

Students who are visually impaired represent the entire range of ability level from profoundly developmentally delayed to gifted and talented. When choosing appropriate programming, both the educational ability and visual ability of students must be considered. While there are some programming needs that are universal to all students who have visual impairments, other programming needs differ depending on the severity of the students' visual impairments and the kinds of educational challenges they face.

This guide has identified four groups of students in order to give general guidelines for the kind of programming for low vision that might be most helpful to each group. Since students with visual impairments represent every point on the continuum of visual abilities as well as the continuum of intellectual abilities, some students will be easily placed within these categories. However, some students whose abilities are on the extremes of these categories will be harder to clearly categorize, and the instructor will need to evaluate how closely this information represents each individual student's needs.

When looking at **ability level,** students could be broadly categorized into two groups:

- **Students who are near, at, or above their developmental level**

- **Students who are significantly developmentally delayed**

When looking at **visual functioning,** students could also be broadly categorized into two groups:

- **Students who use vision as their primary source of sensory information**

- **Students who rely on senses other than vision for their primary source of information**

While some programming needs would be similar for all these students, there are some differences in emphasis that may be helpful to point out before the instructor plans the students' programs.

Programming for Students Who are Near, At, or Above Their Developmental Level

Most of these students would probably be attending regular educational programs for most or all of their school day. See page __ for the curricular areas that may need to be included into the students' programs along with their regular education requirements. They might also need:

- Information about how to recognize and adapt to specific problems that might arise when traveling in the environment

- Information about how and when to ask for assistance, including how to develop positive family support from parents and siblings

- Help to develop a realistic positive self-image as persons with a visual impairment which includes realistic expectations for themselves

- Information about successful strategies for ensuring social integration when the visual impairment interferes

WHEN VISION IS A PRIMARY SOURCE OF SENSORY INFORMATION

Since these students are able to use their vision as their primary source of sensory information, their programming would most likely include the following:

- Instruction in how to use any prescribed low vision devices which would enhance visual performance

- Information on how to decide when it is more convenient to use other senses to enhance or substitute for vision

- Information about non-optical devices and equipment that could enhance performance in school and home

- Information about specific adaptations that could be used in unfavorable environmental conditions, such as inappropriate lighting, glare, distance from the visual target, or information about how to eliminate these unfavorable conditions

Initially, these students may require more support from a certified teacher of students with visual impairments, particularly if they need to learn braille and orientation and mobility. Their programming would most likely include teaching the following:

- Instruction in how to use vision to get important information such as identifying shape cues to recognize people and objects

- Help in determining when vision should be used in academic activities and when braille or other tactual or auditory modifications should be used

- Instruction in how to develop tactual and auditory skills as primary channels of information, and how to integrate them with visual information, or use them as a sole source of information

- Instruction in how to develop smell and taste as auxiliary channels of information

- Instruction in how to use any prescribed low vision devices that would be helpful

- Information about spatial and body relationships which are usually learned from visual observation

WHEN SENSES OTHER THAN VISION ARE THE PRIMARY SOURCE OF INFORMATION

Programming for Students Who are Significantly Developmentally Delayed

Students who have been identified by medical personnel or educational diagnosticians as having significant developmental delays would need a program that addresses the functional needs of the students. It would include instruction in how to perform functional activities in the areas of self-care, play and leisure, and work training. Ideally these activities would be learned within the most appropriate setting and whenever possible they would be taught in the setting where the student would be ultimately performing the activities. Skills that support the successful performance of functional activities also need to be assessed and these skills should be taught within the activities. These might include: skills in communication; cognition; use of vision, hearing, and touch; social emotional development; motor skills; functional academics; personal management; and orientation and mobility. A thorough discussion of this type of programming can be found in *Basic Skills for Community Living: A Curriculum for Students with Multiple Disabilities* (Levack, in press).

WHEN VISION IS A PRIMARY SOURCE OF SENSORY INFORMATION

While this group of students uses vision as a primary resource, they may also use touch, hearing, smell and even taste to confirm information. Educational programming should emphasize fostering greater independence by improving students' visual functioning in everyday activities. The goals for programming for these students would include:

- Instructing students to use their vision in functional tasks

- Identifying when it is appropriate to use vision to look at a task at the "critical moment" for most efficient visual functioning (Goetz & Gee, 1987a, 1987b)

- Identifying environmental modifications that would enhance the students' visual functioning

- Teaching students how to use vision to "read" environmental cues which provide information about distinguishing features in the environment

- Teaching students to use their vision in travel to identify landmarks and travel safely

- Identifying if low vision devices are appropriate, taking into consideration whether a particular student can use and care for it effectively

- Helping students identify how and when to ask for assistance

- Helping students develop a realistic and positive self-image as a person with a visual impairment as well as other impairments, while developing realistic expectations for themselves

- Helping students identify and use successful strategies for social integration.

Since their vision is not strong enough to be their primary source of information, these students rely on touch and hearing with additional help from smell and taste as their primary source of information about their world. If they have any functional vision, it is important to teach them how to use it in efficient ways. The goal for programming for these students would include:

- Helping students to develop their tactual abilities so they can be used with vision whenever possible, but used independently when necessary

- Helping students to develop their auditory abilities so they can be used with vision whenever possible, but used independently when necessary

- Teaching students how to use visual cues to perform more efficiently within specific task training

- Teaching students to use smell and taste for functional information

- Helping the students identify how and when to ask for assistance

- Teaching students to travel independently within familiar routes

- Helping students develop a realistic positive self-image as persons with multiple disabilities, including developing realistic expectations for themselves

- Helping students identify and use successful strategies for social integration when their disabilities interfere

- Providing a meaningful experiential base for the development of symbolic language.

When students have sustained severe brain damage which affects the visual pathways and the visual cortex, they are said to have a cortical visual impairment (Groenveld, Jan & Leader, 1990). These students can have normal eye capacity but once the image reaches the brain the information is not interpreted or processed accurately. Students with cortical visual impairment differ from students who have an impairment in the eye. While students with cortical visual impairments may see an accurate visual image, for some reason they cannot interpret it accurately. On the other hand, students with eye disorders have difficulty obtaining a good visual image, but usually have little or no difficulty processing and interpreting the visual information accurately, once enough information is present. Some students have both cortical visual impairments and eye disorders.

Students with cortical visual impairment need help to successfully decode the visual images that they receive. Some guidelines for helping these students develop their visual efficiency include:

- **Use other sensory cues to stimulate or support the visual information** as it is presented to the student. Encourage exploration by touch; then if the student has not looked at it, ask her to do so.

- **Avoid visual overstimulation** by introducing items one at a time in an uncluttered environment.

- **When using other sensory cues to stimulate visual performance use only one sense at a time.** This will help students integrate information and to make it easier to determine which sense gives the student the most effective information. If a student is given many new objects that have strong visual and tactual qualities as well as produce a unique scent or smell, it is difficult to identify which of these qualities the student is responding to. Once it is clear which sensory qualities give the student the most consistent information, objects that have multiple sensory characteristics can be used.

- Some students will consistently look away from an object in specific tasks and perform the task tactually, deliberately avoiding using their vision. While the cause of this behavior is still unproven, looking away seems to help them complete the task. Therefore, **it would not be helpful, in this instance, to try to teach them to use vision to look at a task at the "critical moment".**

- **Watch for preference in color, shape, size, movement, and field.**

- **Make changes gradually** since processing information is difficult for these students. It is important to build in as much familiarity and predictability as possible. It may be necessary to limit the number of activities and even the number of people who work with a student.

- **Try shaking or moving objects as they are brought into students' line of vision,** when introducing them. Moving objects can sometimes be seen more easily than stationary ones.

- **Determine the best position for students to use their eyes.** Sitting may be the most difficult position for them because they must exert so much energy maintaining the sitting position, that they have little energy or attention left to focus on the visual task.

- **Visual cues should be bold, simple, and consistently used** throughout programming. Generalization can occur more easily when the same visual cues or objects are used in different activities.

- **Present visual stimuli in a simple figure-ground environment.** Avoid visual clutter and maintain high contrast between the background and the object being viewed. Students may bring the object close to their eyes to block out extraneous background information, so they can focus more easily.

Additional information about cortical visual impairment can be found on the chart on page 131.

Caton, H. (Ed.). (1991). *Print and braille literacy: Selecting appropriate learning media.* Louisville, KY: American Printing House for the Blind.

Corn, A. L. (1983). Visual function: A theoretical model for individuals with low vision. *Journal of Visual Impairment and Blindness, 77,* 8, 373-377.

Donaldson, R. & Christiansen, J. (1990). Consultation and collaboration: A decision-making model. *Teaching Exceptional Children, 22,* 2, 22-25.

Downing J. & Bailey, B. R. (1990a). Developing vision use within functional daily activities for students with visual and multiple disabilities. *RE:view, 21,* 4, 209-220.

Downing, J. & Bailey, B. R. (1990b). Sharing the responsibility: Using a transdisciplinary team approach to enhance the learning of students with severe disabilities. *Journal of Educational and Psychological Consultation, 1,* 3, 259.

Educating students with visual impairments: Criteria for exemplary programs. (1991). Austin, TX: Texas Education Agency.

Erin, J. N. (1986). Teachers of the visually handicapped: How can they best serve children with profound handicaps? *Education of the Visually Handicapped, 18,* 1, 15-25.

Erin, J. N. (1988). The teacher-consultant. *Education of the Visually Handicapped, 20,* 2, 57-64.

Erin, J. N. (1989). Cortical visual impairment: Implications for service delivery. *Journal of Vision Rehabilitation, 3,* 4, 1-10.

Goetz, L. & Gee, K. (1987a). Functional vision programming: A model for teaching visual behaviors in natural contexts. In L. Goetz, D. Guess, & K. Stremel-Campbell (Eds.), *Innovative program design for individuals with dual sensory impairments.* Baltimore: Paul Brooks.

Goetz, L. & Gee, K. (1987b). Teaching visual attention in functional contexts: Acquisition and generalization of complex visual motor skills. *Journal of Visual Impairment and Blindness, 81,* 3, 115-117.

Greenblatt, S. L. (1989). *Providing services for people with vision loss: A multidisciplinary perspective.* Lexington, MA: Resources for Rehabilitation.

Groenveld, M., Jan, J. E., & Leader, P. (1990). Observations on the habilitation of children with cortical visual impairment. *Journal of Visual Impairment and Blindness, 84,* 1, 11-15.

Harley, R. K., Garcia, M., & Williams, M. F. (1989). The educational placement of visually impaired children. *Journal of Visual Impairment and Blindness, 83,* 10, 512-516.

Hazekamp, J. & Huebner, K. M. (Eds.). (1989). Appendix E: Position papers, Council for Exceptional Children. In *Program planning and evaluation for blind and students with visual impairments: National guidelines for educational excellence.* New York: American Foundation for the Blind.

Hazekamp, J. & Huebner, K. M. (Eds.). (1989). Planning and providing instructional services. In *Program planning and evaluation for blind and students with visual impairments: National guidelines for educational excellence.* New York: American Foundation for the Blind.

Hazekamp, J. & Huebner, K. M. (Eds.). (1989). Unique educational needs related to a visual impairment. In *Program planning and evaluation for blind and students with visual impairments: National guidelines for educational excellence.* New York: American Foundation for the Blind.

Hofstetter, H. W. (1991). Efficacy of low vision services for visually impaired children. *Journal of Visual Impairment and Blindness, 85,* 1, 20-22.

Horner, R. H., Meyer, L. H., & Fredricks, H. D. (1986). *Education of learners with severe handicaps: Exemplary service strategies.* Baltimore: Paul Brooks.

Koenig, A. J. & Holbrook, M. C. (1989). Determining the reading medium for students with visual impairments: A diagnostic teaching approach. *Journal of Visual Impairment and Blindness, 83,* 6, 296-302.

Koenig, A. J. & Holbrook, M. C. (1991). Determining the reading medium for visually impaired students via diagnostic teaching. *Journal of Visual Impairment and Blindness, 85,* 2, 61-68.

Levack, N. (Ed.). (in press). *Basic skills for community living: A curriculum for students with multiple disabilities.* Austin, TX: Texas School for the Blind and Visually Impaired.

Mangold, S. S. (Ed.). (1982). *A teacher's guide to the special educational needs of blind and visually handicapped children.* New York: American Foundation for the Blind.

Mangold, S. S. & Mangold, P. N. (1989). Selecting the most appropriate primary learning medium for students with functional vision. *Journal of Visual Impairment and Blindness, 83,* 6, 294-296.

Michael, M. G. & Paul, P. V. (1991). Early intervention for infants with deaf-blindness. *Exceptional Children, 1,* 200-209.

Moore, S. (1984). The need for programs and services for visually handicapped infants. *Education for the Visually Handicapped, 15, 2,* 48-55.

Morse, M. T. (1990). Cortical visual impairment in young children with multiple disabilities. *Journal of Visual Impairment and Blindness, 84,* 5, 200-203.

Morse, M. T. (1991). Visual gaze behaviors: Considerations in working with visually impaired multiply handicapped children. *RE:view, 23,* 1, 5-15.

Orelove, F. P. & Sobsey, D. (1987). *Educating children with multiple disabilities: A transdisciplinary approach.* Baltimore: Paul Brooks.

Rogow, S. M. (1988). *Helping the visually impaired child with developmental problems: Effective practice in home, school, and community.* New York: Teacher's College Press.

Tuttle, D. W. (1986). Educational programming. In G. T. Scholl (Ed.), *Foundations of education for blind and visually handicapped children and youth: Theory and practice.* New York: American Foundation for the Blind.

Ward, M. E. (1986). Planning the individualized education program. In G. T. Scholl (Ed.), *Foundations of education for blind and visually handicapped children and youth: Theory and practice.* New York: American Foundation for the Blind.

Zambone, A. (1989). Serving the young child with visual impairments: An overview of disability impact and intervention needs. *Infants and Young Children, 2,* 2, 11-23.

Assessment

The Assessment Process

The process of diagnosing and assessing the functional use of low vision and determining a need for special education services has many steps. Each student's unique needs and abilities will determine which of these steps are appropriate. The process may include:

DETECTION

There are many ways that a suspected visual loss might be detected. Family members or other adults might observe unusual visual behaviors. A vision problem might be detected during a routine medical examination. Or a vision screening conducted by the school or another health agency might indicate a possible vision problem.

VISION SCREENING

Each state has its own system for screening the vision of school-aged children. Vision screening is the routine testing of school-aged children to determine visual acuity, muscle balance and any other readily apparent vision problems. In Texas, the Texas Department of Health trains and certifies anyone who is responsible for vision screening. Further information can be obtained from Vision, Hearing and Speech Services, Texas Department of Health, 1100 West 49th Street,. Austin, TX 78756-3199, (512) 458-7420, or any Texas Department of Health Vision, Hearing and Speech Services Regional Office. They also produce a *Vision Screening Manual: Addendum* (1988) which describes the requirements for vision screening in school programs, gives suggestions for how to use a variety of screening instruments, and offers information about how to interpret the findings. This manual is available after completing the training.

Throughout Texas and the nation, chapters of the Society to Prevent Blindness have volunteer projects to assist with screening the vision of preschool children. Any local chapter can give information about preschool screening and any other projects.

The student with a suspected vision problem should be taken to a licensed eye specialist (i.e., an ophthalmologist or an optometrist). If a visual impairment is diagnosed, low vision devices may be prescribed, medical and/or surgical intervention may be prescribed, or recommendations may be made for the student's educational program.

EXAMINATION
BY AN
EYE SPECIALIST

Once the physical origins and implications of the a visual impairment are identified, an evaluation at a low vision clinic is necessary to determine if optical or non-optical low vision devices would be helpful.

CLINICAL
LOW VISION
EVALUATION

A functional vision assessment must be conducted by a certified teacher of students with visual impairments. The instructor will need to solicit input from the student's family and any others who have information about how the student performs visually.

FUNCTIONAL
VISION
ASSESSMENT

An assessment of the most appropriate learning media must be done annually by a professional who is certified in the education of students who are visually impaired for all students who are school age. This assessment is used to determine eligibility for special education services as a student with a visual impairment, to determine the student's primary learning medium or media and primary literary medium or media, and to determine whether the student is functionally blind.

LEARNING MEDIA
ASSESSMENT

Each step in this process involves professionals with different areas of expertise. This compilation of information is essential for successful educational programming. Each part of this process is described more thoroughly in the following sections.

The Medical Examination and Report

If a student has a suspected or previously diagnosed vision problem, a thorough eye examination should be conducted by a licensed ophthalmologist or optometrist. In Texas, a current eye report must be filed in a student's eligibility folder and appropriate information from this report must be submitted to the Texas Education Agency. The Texas Education Agency has designed a State of Texas Interagency Eye Examination Report which can be used by school districts and all state agencies whenever an ophthalmological or optometric examination is needed. A copy of this form can be found in the Appendix on page 203.

The information contained in the eye report follows the examination and can vary depending on the doctor's examination, the doctor's familiarity with the student, and the student's ability to cooperate. It is helpful when the following information has been included:

- The etiology, medical history, and diagnosis
- Visual acuity, near and distant
- Muscle function
- Intra-ocular pressure (I.O.P.) reading
- Visual field assessment
- Information about color vision
- Information about lighting needs and light sensitivity
- Recommended prescription lenses or low vision devices, if appropriate
- Recommended treatment (e. g., further testing, referral to other specialists, genetic analysis, training, medication, surgery, monitoring), if appropriate
- Precautions or suggestions, if appropriate
- Projected date for follow-up, re-evaluation

Recommendations for braille or large type should not be included on this report. This decision is primarily the responsibility of a certified teacher of students with visual impairments and the education team.

This is not a clinical low vision evaluation. This is a primary care evaluation to determine the presence of a pathological/refractive eye condition and to ascertain the need for medical or surgical intervention to prevent further loss of vision. The clinical low vision evaluation should be conducted once the student is determined to be visually impaired. This should be done in conjunction with other diagnostic services that are being used to determine an appropriate educational program for the student.

In special situations, the following clinical testing procedures may be used to determine extent and type of impairment.

Arteriography: the visualization of arteries by injecting radiopaque material that can be seen by X-ray enhancement.

Computerized Axial Tomography (CAT) or Computerized Tomography (CT): serial sections of the brain (or body) are studied through the use of computerized radiography. This process uses low dosage X-rays and shows fine detail in tissue. It is sensitive to calcification and can identify retinoblastoma, brain abnormalities and optic nerve abnormalities.

Contrast-Sensitivity Function (CSF): a way to test the patient's ability to detect detail which has subtle gradations in grayness between a test target and background. Specially designed targets are printed on cards. In hearing impairments, different decibel losses and differing frequency create differing functional losses of hearing with vision. Low frequency losses create problems with mobility while high frequency losses result in loss of detail vision and often require more light and high contrast materials. Contrast sensitivity tests will elicit these specific types of losses.

Electromyogram (EMG): records the electrical activity of extraocular muscles by inserting needles into those muscles.

Electronystagmogram (ENG): electrical measurement of eye movement.

Electro-oculogram (EOG): records the resting potential of the eye. It is often a supplementary test to the Electroretinogram (ERG). Since this test is more sensitive to the macula, it can help to identify macular degeneration. This test can also measure eye movement, and can measure certain types of nystagmus, but it is a highly specialized technique and the information gained is only useful to a small number of clinicians.

Electroperimetry: computerized visual field testing; electrodes are attached to the scalp which record electrical impulses produced in response to visual stimuli.

Electroretinogram (ERG): measures retinal function after light flashes of varying intensity; tests rod and cone function. This procedure does not measure macular malfunction or optic nerve defects and is widely used in ophthalmic research.

Fluorescein Angiography: a solution of sodium fluorescein is injected into the blood vessels of the arm and is monitored as it is circulated through the eyes. It is used to evaluate the potency of the retinal, choroidal, and iris blood vessels.

Forced-Choice Preferential Looking (FPL) or ***Preferential Looking (PL):*** a subjective evaluation of vision in pre-verbal children. A series of pairs of card targets are presented, one of each pair having a patterned stimulus. Activity is measured by recording which card the child looks at. The target cards have varying widths of lines which approximate acuities.

Optokinetic Drum: a rotating drum, approximately 10" in diameter. The drum is covered with black and white vertical stripes. When rotated slowly (at a distance of about a foot from the patient), the revolving stripes induce a jerky nystagmus if they are able to be seen by the patient. By varying the width of the stripes, the approximate measure of acuity can be estimated in low functioning children.

Ultrasonogram: high frequency, inaudible ultrasound waves are directed into the eye, to detect areas of interference; sound waves penetrate opaque tissues and solid masses (e.g., cataracts). A probe can also be put on the eyelid to show sections or shapes of lesions. The procedure can also delineate the axial length of the eyeball and anterior chamber for intraocular lens calculations. It is also called "diagnostic ultrasound", "echography", and "echo-ophthalmology" and is only used by specialists.

Visually Evoked Response (VER) or ***Visually Evoked Potential (VEP):*** provides a computerized recording of electrical activity at the back of the brain (occipital cortex) which results from light flashes which stimulate the retina. Each eye can be tested separately. It is used to detect defects in the retina-to-brain nerve pathway.

Common Medical Terms

The following terms may be found on the medical report.

↑	increase
↓	decrease
Δ	prism diopter
+	plus or convex lens (the number following the + will be in diopters, the unit of measurement for the lens), corrects farsightedness or hyperopia
—	minus or concave lens (the number following the — will be in diopters, the unit of measurement for the lens), corrects nearsightedness or myopia
A.C.	anterior chamber
add	an additional correction to the corrective lens, usually a bifocal prescription
bil	bilateral
C, C.C.	with correction
C.F.	count fingers, an inaccurate measurement of visual acuity
C.S.M.	central steady and maintained fixation
C.V.F.	central visual field
D	diopter
E	esophoria
E.T.	esotropia
H	hyperphoria
H.M.	hand movements, an inaccurate measurement of visual acuity that implies a student can see the doctor's hand move

H.T.	hypertropia
I.O.L.	intra-ocular lens
I.O.P.	intra-ocular pressure
L. Proj.	light projection
L.P.	light perception
N.L.P.	no light perception; total blindness
N.P.C.	near point convergence
N.V.	near vision
O.D.	oculus dexter (right eye)
O.N.	optic nerve
O.S.	oculus sinister (left eye)
O.U.	oculi uterque (both eyes)
P.D.	prism diopter
P.P.	near point
P.R.	far point
S, S.S., S.C.	sans (without) correction
S.T.	esotropia
V.A.	visual acuity
V.F.	visual field
W.N.L.	within normal limits
X	with a number in front of the X, it refers to the power of a magnifying device
X.T.	exotropia

Visual Acuity - The measurement of the sharpness of vision as it relates to the ability to discriminate detail. It includes distance and near visual acuity with and without correction. An acuity of 20/200 means that this person must stand at 20 feet to see what someone with normal vision can discriminate at 200 feet. This does not mean that the person sees with the same clarity as one with 20/20 acuity, only that he is able to determine separations in detail at that distance.

Lenses - The lenses prescribed can tell a great deal about an individual's eye condition. The stronger the lens, the poorer the uncorrected vision. However, thick glasses do not mean that a person is necessarily corrected to within "normal" levels of vision. In addition, glasses cannot correct all types of visual impairments, and getting stronger glasses is not a solution for many people with low vision.

- A **convex, or plus lens,** which converges light rays, tends to increase the size of an image received. A plus lens may also be used to direct light rays entering the eye so that they come to a focus on, rather than behind the retina of the eye. Lens power greater than +12D may mean that the student has no crystalline lens inside his eye, because of cataract surgery resulting in *aphakia*, or it may mean that she is extremely farsighted.

- A **concave, or minus lens,** which diverges light rays, tends to decrease the size of the image received. A minus lens can also be used to converge light rays so that they focus on the retina rather than in front of it. A very strong minus lens, such as -6D to -8D indicates extreme nearsightedness, which is also referred to as *high myopia.*

- In case of a **large disparity between the lenses** (anisometropia) for each eye, a student may tend to favor one eye over the other, depending on the task.

- It is important for students with **astigmatism (an irregular curvature** in the cornea corrected by cylindrical lenses) not only to wear the lenses at all times, but to keep them properly adjusted on their face.

Field of vision - An illustration on the eye report is often used to indicate any restrictions in the field of vision. It is possible to have good central vision with limited peripheral vision, to have good peripheral vision with limited central vision, and to have scattered field vision. Each eye may have different patterns of field vision loss. Such students may need to learn to direct their gaze differently, and will appear not to look at an object directly. This is called eccentric viewing. They may also need to learn how to optimize the visual field they do have or to use environmental cues to detect the presence of people or objects.

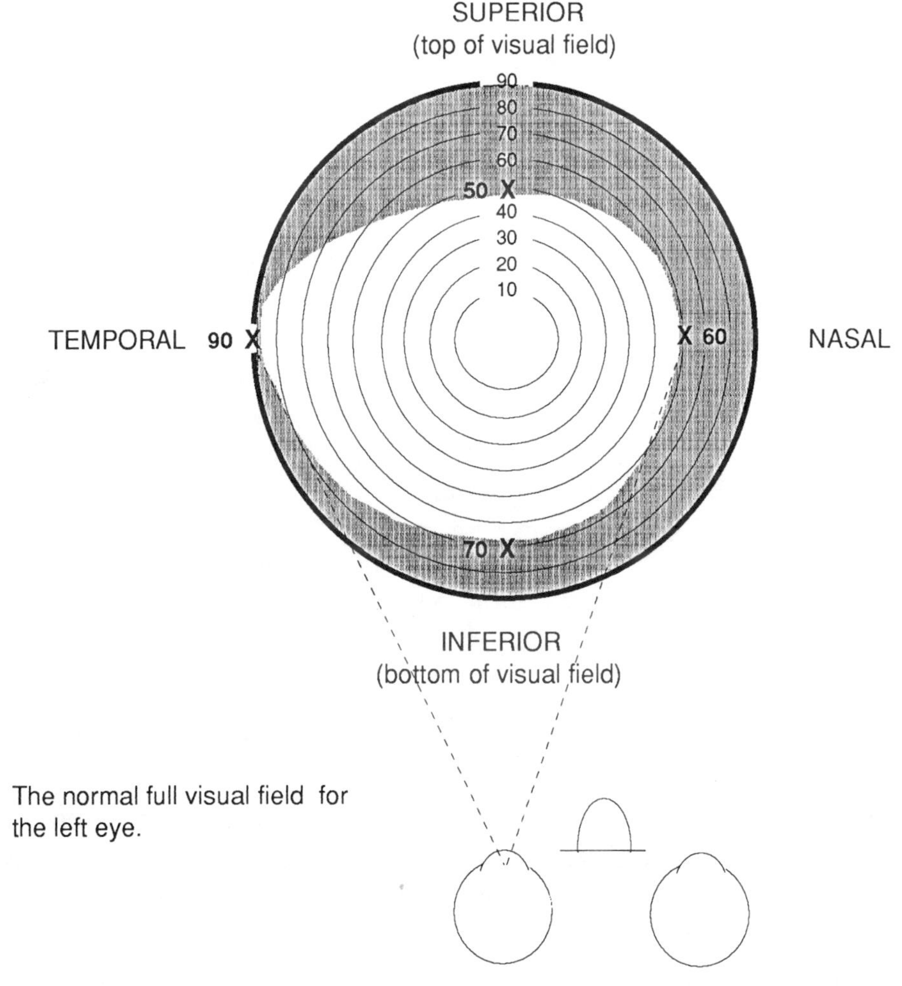

Source: Jose, R. (1983). *Understanding low vision,* p. 98. New York: American Foundation for the Blind.

Special Considerations for
Successful Examinations

WHEN THE STUDENTS ARE YOUNG OR HAVE DEVELOPMENTAL DISABILITIES

Young children and students who are developmentally delayed may need additional support to help the examiner to obtain meaningful information. Children should always be accompanied by someone who can give the doctor accurate information about their visual performance. In addition to a parent, a VH instructor might also attend.

When students can understand the tasks that they will be asked to do in the doctor's office, it is helpful to preview and teach in advance the tasks that will be asked of them at the exam (e. g., pointing, matching pictures or placing a hand on a picture of a hand). Talk about how important it is to sit in the examining chair and be still while a light is shined in their eyes, or when objects are brought close to their eyes. These desired behaviors can be practiced in advance. The doctor can be consulted prior to the exam to determine what kinds of assessment materials will be used and whether to show these materials to the students in advance so they can practice labeling or matching them.

A clinical low vision evaluation of infants and severely delayed students who have no formal communication skills is more difficult. Parents and VH instructors can give the doctor important information for diagnosis by performing a careful functional vision assessment before the examination and reporting their findings to the doctor. Often a familiar person who accompanies the student to the examination can assist by modeling, interpreting, prompting, reassuring, physically assisting, or reinforcing the desired responses (Cress, Spellman, De Briere, Sizemore, Northam, & Johnson, 1981). Adapted tests that rely on matching or pointing may be helpful as they do not require a verbal response. Diagnostic procedures, such as Forced Choice Preferential Looking (FPL), Preferential Looking (PL), or Optokinetic Drum may also be helpful. These procedures have been described on page 27. As much as possible, students should be prepared in advance for these procedures.

Positioning can have a strong impact on the alert state and the students' overall ability to respond. This is particularly true for students who have severe multiple disabilities.

For these students it is possible that the exam will only be able to produce a diagnosis. A thorough functional vision assessment is also needed to provide teachers, therapists and parents with the most useful information about the students' needs.

As a last resort in rare cases when the student is able to give minimal cooperation, some level of sedation may be needed. This should be determined by the eye care specialist.

Students will need to be taught from an early age how to communicate with the doctor to give the kinds of responses that help the doctor to make accurate diagnoses, and to ask the questions that help them understand their own condition. Parents and teachers can model good communication skills when the student is young as they work with the doctor to give accurate information and ask pertinent questions. As the students grow, parents and teachers can talk to students before the examination to help them identify what questions or concerns they might want to bring up. If needed, the students can role play or practice asking these questions.

To be sure that nothing is forgotten, the questions can be written out in advance and brought to the exam. Some sample questions that might be asked include:

"Will my vision ever get better?"

"What can be done so that I can see better?"

"Is there another specialist whom I should see?"

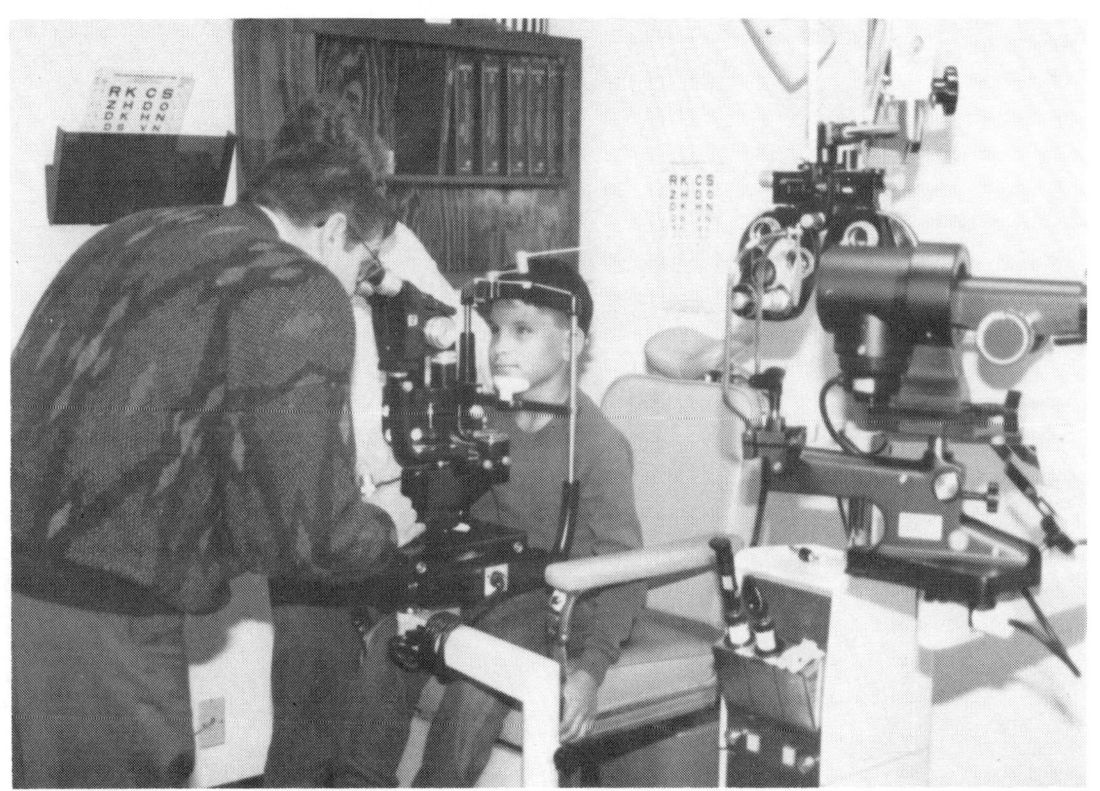

Ophthalmologists or optometrists perform clinical low vision evaluations. This evaluation assesses the students' potential to function visually and determines if low vision devices and services can be prescribed to improve the students' use of vision in everyday life. It is very helpful when the Functional Vision Assessment precedes the student's visit to the low vision clinic. As with the medical examination, it is helpful if a teacher can attend this evaluation as well as the students' parents, whenever possible.

A clinical low vision evaluation should review any devices that students are currently using. Information should be gathered about any visual tasks the students want or need to do that are currently difficult or in need of improvement. The students and clinic staff can then evaluate what devices or adapted techniques might be helpful. Finally, students may need a trial period with training to determine which devices or techniques are useful. The clinical evaluation should address the students' case history, ocular health, acuities, fields, color vision, refraction, binocular vision, and magnification (Jose, 1983). A thorough discussion of this evaluation can be found in "Clinical Examination of Visually Impaired Individuals" in *Understanding Low Vision* (Jose, 1983, chap. 8).

Students who have multiple impairments may benefit from a low vision evaluation, even if they cannot use a low vision device. Low vision clinicians can often provide more information about their visual functioning than has been included on the eye report, particularly if "blind" or "untestable" was the only description of the visual functioning on the report.

Two very important parts of the clinical low vision evaluation are the follow up visits and the application in the students' daily activities.

A list of low vision centers where these services are available can be found in the *American Foundation for the Blind Directory of Services for Blind and Visually Impaired Persons in the United States* (1988). In addition, some private practitioners with a low vision specialty are able to provide low vision clinical evaluations. Local ophthalmologists and optometrists can be contacted to find out where this service is locally available. However, these local services usually do not include a multidisciplinary approach.

A functional vision assessment offers an organized plan for observing how the students use their vision to perform routine tasks. Langley (1980, p. 9) says that a functional vision assessment serves the following purposes:

• To assess a student's vision to determine whether a visual impairment is interfering with the learning process.

• To enable the teachers and other personnel to determine the quantity and quality of a student's functional vision. This information can then be used to plan intervention strategies which maximize the student's potential to use her vision purposefully.

Once the functional vision assessment has been completed, a report should be written, shared with the parents and primary people who work with the student and placed in the student's file. It should be written in clear simple terms that can be understood by any lay person and should include:

- The student's name, date of birth, school, grade or placement

- The evaluator's name and title or credentials

- Whether the student has been determined to meet eligibility criteria for visually handicapped students according to agency and/or state rules

- Diagnosis of the visual impairment, as found in the medical report

- A summary of the ophthalmologist's and/or optometrist's reports

- A list of other significant impairments

- A list of medications being taken, and whether they affect visual functioning

- A synopsis of the findings from the functional vision assessment

- Recommendations for programming, with specific recommendations for additional services, adaptations, and teaching methods

- Translation of the student's eye condition into practical language (Jose, 1983).

Ideally, this information can be taken from the functional vision assessment form and translated into a concise report with little difficulty. It should contain information which can be used for the development of a program for using low vision, as well as information which will assist the student in his classroom and outdoor activities.

Assessing Students Who are Very Young or Who Have Significant Developmental Disabilities

When working with children who are very young and students who have significant developmental delays, particularly when they do not have effective communication skills. Careful observation is essential. The following suggestions may be helpful:

- **Review developmental testing** that has been done to get an idea of where a student is functioning in order to choose materials that are appropriate.

- **Observe the students in a variety of familiar situations** performing routine tasks or activities.

- **Find out what motivates the students to look.** Use objects and activities similar to those that have been motivating in the past.

- **Be sure that the students are physically stable, comfortable, sufficiently alert,** and positioned to maximize visual field and eye muscle movements. Note students' responses in different positions (e.g., sidelying, supine, sitting).

- **Try to develop a rapport with the student before assessing**, or ask a person who has this rapport to work with the student while you observe.

- When **two people evaluate together**, one can administer the assessment items while the other closely observes for subtle indications of visual performance or changes in behavior (Langley, 1980).

- Recognize that you may be able to observe only visual attending and visual examining behaviors, so it will be important to **get as much specific information as possible from these activities** (e. g., size, color, shape of object preferred, lighting preferred, student's best position for visual attention, preferred field).

- **Observe what senses are used first when given a new object.** Is it touched, looked at, or put it in the mouth? Do the students listen to the sound that it makes?

- **Observe where objects are held to look at them.**

- If a student is not verbal or is severely motorically impaired, **responses may be subtle.** Look for changes in students' eyes such as widening, squinting, tearing, or movement, as well as increased or decreased body movement, changes in breathing, or behaviors which are either quieting or exciting.

- **Look for any signs of visual behaviors** such as light flicking using a hand or objects, mouth opening when objects are near, or avoidance of a visual stimulus.

- **The students may need additional time to respond.** Go slowly. It may take several trials with the same object before a response is made.

- **The students may perform better during several short sessions** than one long session.

- **Use a variety of objects,** but not so many that students are overwhelmed. Change them occasionally to prevent boredom.

- **Introduce objects that have only visual properties at first.** If students do not respond, add either auditory, tactual and olfactory cues. Or, if students are reluctant to look, establish a game of sorting or matching with three dimensional shapes, and when the students have understood the task, substitute with pictures or two dimensional shapes.

- When the student does not respond immediately, **vary the situation.** Try changing the lighting. Change the size, color, or contrast of the object, or change the object itself. Try changing the position of the student.

- If students seem to respond best to other sensory stimulation (e.g., auditory, tactual, olfactory), **pair the visual stimulation with the preferred sensory stimulation** to see if a visual response can be trained.

A suggested functional vision assessment form has been included in the appendix on pages 205 to 216 for duplication. There are many functional vision assessment forms that ask students to perform visual tasks in isolation. This assessment is slightly different because it is based on observing a student perform routine activities and watching for specific visual abilities. It recommends making adaptations at the time of the assessment to see how the student's visual abilities can be enhanced, and then recording the observations and making recommendations for programming. It is hoped that this approach will help the instructor to identify the activities that are most functional and effective for teaching the student skills in enhancing visual performance. If this assessment form is not preferred, a list of other functional vision assessments can be found on pages 55 and 56.

I. Medical History

- Review the student's medical reports for pertinent information including: age of onset, any diagnosed conditions or diseases, any surgeries or other medical interventions, a description of the student's eye which includes any anomalies, the student's visual acuity in each eye and in both eyes together, any identified field loss, the prognosis for the student's condition, any medications the student is now taking or restrictions on activity, and any family history of visual impairments.

- On the next line write the official diagnosis or diagnoses.

- If the reports have mentioned other significant impairments (e.g., diagnosis of developmental disabilities, motor impairments), list them on the next line.

II. General Observations

- This section should include information about how the student is functioning in the overall environment.

- It could include information about interactions with peers and adults, what is motivating to him, and any information about his family or school situation which may have implications for his visual functioning.

III. Observations of the Student in Familiar Near Vision Tasks

- In order to evaluate how the student is using his vision, it is helpful to observe him performing familiar tasks that require near vision (16 inches or less). If you have difficulty identifying which tasks to evaluate, talk to the student's other teachers and family for ideas. These activities can include eating; dressing; brushing teeth; using regular print textbooks, workbooks, paper and rulers; putting objects in a container; using communication boards; sorting objects; looking at a toy; putting objects away; doing laundry; cooking; or finding a radio or television channel.

- Once the activity has been chosen, observe the student to see whether vision is used. Does he look at an object (visual attending) or look at the object carefully for details (visual exploring) or look while reaching for it (visually guided motor behaviors)? Write this in the second column.

- Observe whether he looks continually or only during the critical moment. If he is not looking, try to identify the critical moment for looking during that task to plan when prompting might be appropriate (Goetz & Gee, 1987a, 1987b).

- In the third column, describe the environmental conditions that prevail, such as the type of lighting, the size of the objects used, the type of background and the distance between the object and the student.

- If the student is not using his vision, try some adaptations and interventions to see if enhancing the visual image or changing the environmental conditions might help. These adaptations might include changing the lighting, varying the color, contrast, size or arrangement of the object(s), pairing an auditory or tactual prompt or cue, or using a low vision device such as a magnifier. The chart on eye conditions on pages 114 through 148 has general recommendations for adaptations related to specific eye conditions and may be helpful as a place to start. When you have found successful adaptations, write them in the last column.

- Before completing this section, decide how many near vision tasks to observe. If the student's visual performance is consistent, it may only need to be two or three. However, if the student's performance is inconsistent, many more activities may need to be observed at different times before getting a sense of what conditions are helpful and what ones are not.

- When this side of the chart is completed, turn it over to answer the general questions about the student's performance on near vision tasks. It is hoped that this latter section will help clarify how the student is performing and identify whether there are specific visual abilities that should be targeted for instruction.

IV. Observations of Students in Familiar Intermediate and Distance Vision Tasks

- While some students will not be able to perform tasks at the distances in this section, it is important to determine the maximum distance that the student can see under specific conditions such as size of objects and amount and type of lighting in the environment.

- First, choose several activities at intermediate distances (16 inches to three feet) and then try distances beyond three feet. Be sure to use activities that are motivating to the student. The following activities are examples of how the student may be using his intermediate and distance vision: looking at a familiar person as they enter the room, locating an exit in a room, avoiding objects while moving around a room, retrieving a toy, visually following a silent pull toy or pet, recognizing familiar people, watching television or movies, identifying pictures or decorations on the wall, locating familiar equipment on a playground, recognizing a bus as it approaches, or finding a crosswalk.

- Follow the same procedures for observation as you did in the near vision tasks.

V. Academic Considerations

- If the student is able to perform academic tasks such as reading and writing, or is attending general education academic
classes that follow standard teaching techniques such as use
of the blackboard and demonstrations at the front of the class,
or if the student uses electronic equipment such as computers,
or electronic reading systems, it is important to fill out as much
of this section as applies to the student.

VI. Environmental Conditions

- Based on your observations of the student during the preced-
ing visual tasks, answer the questions in this section which give
information about how the student performs under different
environmental conditions.

VII. Visual Acuity

- While it may not be possible to obtain a visual acuity for all
students, when possible it is important to compare the acuities
that have been recorded on medical reports with informal visual
acuities obtained when the student is performing in a familiar
setting. Information about instruments that can be used to test
visual acuity can be found in the Appendix on pages 229 to
232.

- Since this is an assessment of functional vision, students may
wear corrective lenses during acuity testing and testing need
only be done for both eyes together (O.U.). Students may also
be assessed with and without the use of prescribed optical
devices.

VIII. Recommendations

- This section includes information that can be helpful in writing
the functional vision report as well as planning further
assessment, evaluation and programming. It may be particularly useful in IEP development. Simply fill in the answers.

WHAT IT IS

An important component in any assessment for students who are visually impaired is determining what are the most efficient learning media for the student. The learning media is defined as the materials or methods that students use in conjunction with the sensory channels to get information. Examples of visual learning media would include pictures, charts, diagrams, video, modeling, imitation and demonstrations. Tactual learning media would include real objects; hand-over-hand modeling; physical prompting; full size or scale models; tactual charts, diagrams, and maps. Auditory learning media would include verbal descriptions, conversation, taped materials, environmental sounds, verbal guidance, class discussion, and lectures.

It is also necessary to assess what is the most efficient literary medium. The literary medium is a subset or component of the learning media and is based on what sensory channels the student will use for reading and writing. This would include print if the student used vision and braille if the student used touch.

It is important to keep in mind that many students use more than one learning medium as well as more than one literary medium. Students can have primary and secondary learning and literary media. The primary learning medium is the medium most frequently used during classroom instruction, which can be utilized in a wide variety of settings inside and outside the classroom, and should permit both reading and writing (Mangold & Mangold, 1989). Students who have functional vision often use a secondary learning medium to perform tasks that are not easily performed in the primary medium. This secondary medium can also alleviate fatigue experienced when using the primary medium over long periods of time (Mangold & Mangold, 1989).

In Texas, a learning media assessment is required as part of the comprehensive assessment for any student who is suspected of having a visual impairment. This is to be done by a professional certified in the education of students with visual impairments. Together with information from the students' eye examination, and the functional vision assessment, the findings from this learning media assessment are used to

- determine eligibility for special education services as a student with a visual impairment

- determine the student's primary learning media and primary literacy medium

- determine whether the student is functionally blind.

The decision on the literacy medium or media is made at the Admission, Review and Dismissal (ARD) committee meeting. If the committee feels that the evidence for determining the literary medium is inconclusive, they may recommend ongoing assessment; however, a date must be scheduled to reconvene to make this decision. If the student is a prereader or a nonreader and a decision about the student's literary medium cannot be made at that time, recommendations should be made on the student's general learning media. This might include suggestions such as pairing physical and verbal prompts during instruction, using bold visual cues on familiar objects to attract the student's attention or adding tactual cues to objects that the student uses frequently.

When a student is identified as visually impaired, the IEP must specify

- the student's primary learning medium or media based on the assessment results

- the recommendations for use of visual, tactual, and auditory learning media.

WHEN A STUDENT IS DETERMINED TO BE FUNCTIONALLY BLIND

In Texas, if it is determined that the student will use tactual media (which includes braille) as a primary tool for learning to be able to communicate in both reading and writing at the same level of proficiency as other students of comparable ability, he is considered to be functionally blind and additional documentation is required:

- the IEP must document the student's strengths and weaknesses in braille skills. For a student who is a prereader or nonreader, this should include information about his strengths or weaknesses in using tactual learning media and whether pre-readiness or readiness level skills should be included in the student's program.

- Each member of the ARD committee must receive information describing the benefits of braille instruction.

- If it is determined that braille instruction is needed, it must be documented that this will be provided by a teacher certified to teach students with visual impairments.

While the learning assessment must be a part of the comprehensive assessment every three years, it should be updated each year as part of the annual IEP reevaluation process. Information about arrangement for instruction specific to braille and/or print, training to compensate for visual loss, and access to special media, tools, appliances, aides, or devices should be provided in this update.

Decisions must always be based on the assessed needs of the student, never on the extraneous logistical factors such as the availability of a teacher certified in the instruction of students with visual impairments, administration convenience or fiscal considerations.

The following guidelines have been proposed to help those making decisions about the selection of a learning medium/media for students who are visually impaired (Caton, 1991, pp. 17-19):

- All visually impaired children have **individual needs** which can vary in relation to specific characteristics.
- Visually impaired children must use **all sensory channels for input in learning** to explore and interact with the environment for gathering and using information.
- A variety of **discrimination and recognition activities** designed for all functional sensory channels is critical, particularly during the readiness period.
- Low vision children must have **functional vision assessments**, at least annually.
- Some children prefer **visual or tactual learning** at an early age, while others may give no indication of a **preference**.
- Blind children and those with profound visual disability **must be given the opportunity to learn braille.**
- Some low vision students may **utilize both braille and print** for selected purposes.
- Many children with moderate visual disability will use print with or without **optical devices.**
- Some low vision students benefit from both braille and print materials until **proficiency** is demonstrated **in a dominant medium.**
- Ongoing **exposure to technology** will help develop literacy skills.
- Some low vision students may learn to write **cursive more easily than manuscript,** first at a chalkboard (gross motor) then at a desk (fine motor).
- **Consider a variety of factors in making decisions,** such as physical and visual fatigue, expenditure of energy and stamina, distance from the page, quantity of reading and writing required, portability of devices, equipment and books, size of print, and availability of optical devices.
- **Use of slate and stylus** is important for blind students.
- **Keyboarding and auditory materials** are valuable supplements.
- **Flexibility** is the key to the use of all types of media for maximum literacy.

Genetic Counseling

Some of the eye conditions that cause visual impairment are inherited. The families of the students, as well as the students themselves, if they are old enough to be interested, may need to meet with genetic counselors to identify whether the condition is inherited or caused by disease or environmental factors. The genetic counselor can give information about the probability of the condition occurring in other members of the family or in the students' own children. Other reasons for genetic counselling include identifying or confirming the diagnosis of an eye disorder which has profound implications for an individual's general health and prognosis.

Although steps in the process of genetic counselling may vary depending on the policy of a particular doctor or clinic, generally the process is as follows:

- **Physicians** (e.g., neonatologists, ophthalmologists, pediatricians) usually **recommend genetic counseling to parents** when they first suspect an inherited disorder.
  or
  Family members discuss their concerns with a physician when there are questions about a particular congenital impairment or disability. If it is suspected that the condition is inherited, the physician may refer them to a genetic clinic, or they may make the initial contact themselves.

- **Medical records for the person with the condition, and sometimes records of other members of the family need to be sent to the clinic as requested.** The counselor or a doctor at the clinic takes a social and genetic history of the family preferably for two or more generations. This is called a "family pedigree" .

- **A physical examination may involve one or more members of the family and diagnostic tests may be prescribed.** These may include blood or tissue samples, a CT (computerized tomography), a CAT (computerized axial tomography), or an amniocentesis if the patient is pregnant.

- **Finally, there should be a counselling session in which the condition can be explained and defined.** Opportunity is provided for the involved persons to ask any questions about the condition and express their feelings. At this time referrals may be made for other social or medical services needed which relate to treatment of the condition.

- **A follow up letter summarizing the findings and the diagnosis should be sent** to the individual and/or the parents or guardian which explains the results of the evaluation.

Instructors may tend to believe that any learning difficulties that students with visual impairments have are a result of their visual impairment. However, students with visual impairments should learn at a rate similar to their unimpaired peers, if their materials and environment have been adapted for their impairment, and they have had the experiences that are prerequisites for the skills or concepts that they are learning. If students are not making adequate progress when all of these conditions have been met the possibility of a learning disability should be considered.

A student can be considered to have a learning disability if there is a significant disorder in the acquisition and use of listening, speaking, reading, writing, reasoning, or mathematical abilities. This disorder is intrinsic to the individual and not caused by educational deprivation, cultural differences, or emotional factors, and is presumed to be due to central nervous system dysfunction and not the result of sensory impairments. (Myers & Hammill, 1990). Students who are visually impaired are not excluded from this definition, but they cannot be considered learning disabled if the problems are primarily the result of their visual impairment.

There are certain characteristics that can be warning signs that a learning disability could be present. None of these characteristics in isolation confirms the presence of a learning disability, and a student may demonstrate some of these characteristics without having a learning disability. However, if a student demonstrates several of these characteristics and is not making progress in school, it may be helpful to contact a teacher of students with learning disabilities and/or a diagnostician for further assessment. These characteristics include:

- **Organic brain dysfunction has been identified** in the students' medical records.

- **Language development is delayed**, especially expressive language.

- **Academic achievement is less than expected.** Despite normal or above normal intelligence and good reasoning skills, the student is unable to achieve in reading, math, and/or writing.

- **The student is highly distractible and there is a lack of organizational skills.** This may include an inability to pay attention, follow oral or written directions, to remember sequences of events, or to keep up with assignments.

- **The student employs avoidance behaviors** such as:

  ❑ Passivity, the student is usually quiet and does not complete assignments or turn in work.

  ❑ Excessive talking which results in assignments not being completed.

  ❑ Blaming the inability to complete a task on the visual impairment. Here, of course, it is important for the teacher to make sure the student's learning environment and materials are adapted for the visual impairment.

  ❑ Blaming the inability to complete work on physical discomfort or fatigue. The student should be evaluated to check for an underlying cause of discomfort or fatigue.

  ❑ General lack of effort or concentration.
  (Harley, Truan, & Sanford, 1987)

- **The learning problem can be remediated** by using different methods of teaching. The student will still have the underlying problem (e. g., difficulties with spatial organization) but can learn to circumvent it.

- **Learning in some areas occurs quickly.** Once teaching methods are matched to the student's learning style, academic improvement becomes evident.

Seven specific areas have been identified (Harley, Truan, & Sanford, 1987) where students who are visually impaired are likely to have learning disabilities: These are:

- ❏ memory (rote memory and logical memory)
- ❏ perception
- ❏ organization
- ❏ concrete learning
- ❏ perseveration and fixation
- ❏ generalization
- ❏ language

It becomes the instructor's task to determine if learning problems are caused by visual images being received and if they can be alleviated by using the teaching methods and adaptations designed to teach students who are visually impaired or whether the learning problems are caused by visual perceptual impairments. If the latter is the case, a referral should be made to an instructor with a specialty in learning disabilities. Working together a determination may be made as to whether methods designed to teach students who are learning disabled would best serve the student. This determination is essential for selecting materials and teaching techniques to be used with students with visual impairments who also have learning disabilities. A discussion of suggested adaptation for students who have learning disabilities can be found on pages 99 and 100.

Barraga, N. C. & Erin, J. N. (1992). Assessment and evaluation of individual functioning. In *Visual handicaps and learning* (3rd ed.). Austin, TX: ProEd.

Brown, C. J. & Langley, M. B. (1984). *Diagnostic/prescriptive model for training inter-disciplinary personnel working with profoundly mentally handicapped learners.* Tallahassee, FL: Department of Education, Bureau of Education for Exceptional Students.

Cassin, B. & Solomon, S. (1990). *Dictionary of eye terminology* (2nd ed.). Gainesville, FL: Triad.

Caton, H. (Ed.). (1991). *Print and braille literacy: Selecting appropriate learning media.* Louisville, KY: American Printing House for the Blind.

Cress, P. J., Spellman, C. R., DeBriere, T. J., Siemore, A. C., Northam, J. K., & Johnson, J. L. (1981). Vision screening for persons with severe handicaps. *TASH Journal, 6,* 41-50.

Educating students with visual impairments: Criteria for exemplary programs. (1991). Austin, TX: Texas Education Agency.

Gittenger, J. & Asdourian, G. (1988). *Manual of clinical problems in ophthalmology.* Boston: Little, Brown.

Greenblatt, S. L. (Ed.). (1989). *Providing services for people with vision loss: A multidisciplinary perspective.* Lexington, MA: Resources for Rehabilitation.

Harley, R. K., Truan, M. B., & Sanford, L. N. (1987). Identifying visually impaired students with learning problems. In *Communication skills for visually impaired learners.* Springfield, IL: Charles Thomas.

Hazekamp, J. & Huebner, K. M. (Ed.). (1989). Appendix D: Assessing vision/low vision. In *Planning and evaluation for blind and students with visual impairments: National guidelines for educational excellence.* New York: American Foundation for the Blind.

Koenig, A. J. & Holbrook, M. C. (1989). Determining the reading medium for students with visual impairments: A diagnostic teaching approach. *Journal of Visual Impairment and Blindness, 83,* 6, 296-302.

Koenig, A. J. & Holbrook, M. C. (1991). Determining the reading medium for visually impaired students via diagnostic teaching. *Journal of Visual Impairment and Blindness, 85,* 2, 61-68.

Koenig, A. J. & Ross, D. B. (1991). A procedure to evaluate the relative effectiveness of reading in large and regular print. *Journal of Visual Impairment and Blindness, 85,* 5, 198-204.

Mangold, S. & Mangold, P. (1989). Selecting the most appropriate primary learning medium for students with functional vision. *Journal of Visual Impairment and Blindness, 83,* 6, 294-296.

Morris, O. F. (1981). Teacher assessment of visual functioning. *Education of the Visually Handicapped, 13,* 2, 42-50.

Myers, P. I. & Hammill, D. D. (1990). *Learning disabilities: Basic concepts, assessment practices, and instructional strategies* (4th ed.). Austin, TX: ProEd.

Orel-Bixler, D., Haegerstrom-Portnoy, G., & Hall, A. (1989). Visual assessment of the multiply handicapped patient. *Optometry and Vision Science, 66,* 8, 530-536.

Pavan-Langston, D. (1985). *Manual of ocular diagnosis and therapy* (2nd ed.). Boston: Little, Brown.

Rex, E. J. (1989). Issues related to literacy of legally blind learners. *Journal of Visual Impairment and Blindness, 77,* 1, 8-11.

Silberman, R. K. & Sowell, V. (1987). The visually impaired student with learning disabilities: Strategies for success in language arts. *Education of the Visually Handicapped, 18,* 4, 139-150.

Stein, H., Slatt, B., & Cook, P. (1982). *Manual of ophthalmic terminology.* St. Louis: C. V. Mosby.

Szlyk, J. P., Arditi, A., Coffey Bucci, P., & Laderman, D. (1990). Self-report in functional assessment of low vision. *Journal of Visual Impairment and Blindness, 84,* 2, 61-66.

Vaughan, D. & Ashbury, T. (1980). *General ophthalmology* (9th ed.). Los Altos, CA: Lang Medical.

Yeadon, A. (Ed.). *International low vision directory.* Philadelphia: Institute for the Visually Impaired, Pennsylvania College of Optometry.

Barraga, N. & Morris, J. E. (1980). Low vision observation checklist and diagnostic assessment procedure. In *Program to develop efficiency in visual functioning.* Louisville, KY: American Printing House for the Blind.

Bishop, V. (1988). Making choices in functional vision evaluations: "Noodles, needles, and haystacks". *Journal of Visual Impairment and Blindness, 82,* 3, 94-99.

Copeland, D., James, P., Richey, K., Seitz, W., & King, P. (1991). *Functional vision evaluation for elementary, secondary blind or visually impaired.* Mt. Pleasant, TX: Region VII Education Service Center.

Functional vision evaluation for the academic student. (n. d.). Midland, TX: Region 18 Education Service Center.

Hall, A., Orel-Bixler, D., & Haegerstrom-Portnoy, G. (1991). Special visual assessment techniques for multiply handicapped persons. *Journal of Visual Impairment and Blindness 85,* 1, 23-29.

Hazekamp, J., & Huebner, K. M. (1989). Appendix D: Functional vision checklist summary sheet (pp. 68-69). In *Program planning and evaluation for blind and students with visual impairments: National guidelines for educational excellence.* New York: American Foundation for the Blind.

Jose, R. T. (Ed.). (1983). Assessment of children with low vision. In *Understanding low vision.* New York: American Foundation for the Blind.

Mangold, S. (1982). The functional vision checklist summary sheet. In *A teacher's guide to the special educational needs of blind and visually handicapped children.* New York: American Foundation for the Blind.

Resource manual for functional vision evaluation. (1984). Austin, TX: Texas Education Agency.

FUNCTIONAL VISION ASSESSMENTS DESIGNED FOR STUDENTS WHO ARE MULTIPLY IMPAIRED

Copeland, D., James, P., Richey, K., Seitz, W., & King, P. (1991). *Functional vision evaluation for infants, severe, profoundly handicapped, and multihandicapped.* Mt. Pleasant, TX: Region VIII Education Service Center.

Efron, M., & DuBoff, B. R. (1975). Appendix C: Teacher's guide for evaluating visual functioning. In *A vision guide for teachers of deaf-blind children.* Raleigh, NC: South Atlantic Regional Center for Services to Deaf-Blind Children.

Erhardt, R. P. (1989). Erhardt developmental vision assessment (EDVA). In *Developmental visual dysfunction: Models for assessment and management.* Tuscon, AR: Therapy Skill Builders.

Functional vision evaluation for the multihandicapped/non-academic/ nonverbal and/or 0-3 year old visually impaired child. (n. d.). Midland, TX: Region 18 Education Service Center.

Jose, R. T. (Ed.). (1989). Assessment of multiply handicapped people. In *Understanding low vision.* New York: American Foundation for the Blind.

Jose, R. T., Smith, A. J., & Shane, K. G. (1980). Evaluating and stimulating vision in the multiply impaired. *Journal of Visual Impairment and Blindness, 74,* 1, 5-21.

Langley, B. (1980). Functional vision inventory for the multiply and severely handicapped. *The New Outlook for the Blind, 70,* 8, 346-350.

Langley, B. (in press). *PAVE.* Louisville, KY: American Printing House for the Blind.

Sailor, W., Utley, B., Goetz, L., Gee, K. J. Baldwin, M., Hatlen, P., & Peterson, J. (1980). *Vision assessment and program manual.* San Francisco: Bay Area Severely Handicapped Deaf Blind Project, San Francisco State University.

Smith A. J. & Cote, K. S. (1982). *Look at me: A resource manual for the development of residual vision in multiply impaired children.* Philadelphia: Pennsylvania College of Optometry Press.

Planning, Teaching and Evaluation

- **Teaching techniques to enhance vision should not be taught in isolation.** Look at what are the particular needs and activities of the students in school and in their everyday life that are affected by their visual performance, and teach to those tasks.

- **Analyze the tasks for what parts are dependent upon vision** and **decide what might make for greater efficiency** in performing them.

- Look for any **adaptations that would make it easier to do the task.** A thorough discussion of adaptations can be found in the next chapter on pages 70 to 100.

- Review the students' IEP and **evaluate what visual skills and adaptations will be needed to address the designated goals and objectives.**

- **Identify any new objectives that should be added** in teaching the use of low vision.

- If students cannot understand or perform the whole task, **consider whether partial participation is an option.** This is often used with students who have severe or multiple impairments. The students team up with another person and share responsibility for doing the task. The parts of the task that cannot be done by the student are done by the partner.

- When choosing tasks and skills to be taught, **consider whether the independence that the students gain justifies time that it will take.** If there are other more important demands on the students' time, compromise may need to be made, or priorities may need to be reevaluated. **The instructor, parent, and the student, whenever possible, will need to decide what is the best use of the student's time.**

Once the needs have been identified, it is necessary to **plan how to implement the programming.** The remainder of this chapter suggests how this can be done.

Three types of instructional approach to enhance visual functioning have been identified by Hall and Bailey (1989). They are *visual environment management*, *visual skills training* and *visually dependent task training*.

VISUAL ENVIRONMENT MANAGEMENT

The instructor applies knowledge about visual development and effective use of adaptations to create an environment or activity that offers opportunities for students to have successful visual experiences that will in turn provide motivation for further looking and use of vision. Specific environments can be designed to encourage particular visual behaviors such as attending, examining, and visually guided motor behaviors. The objects and tasks themselves need to be motivating and reinforcing enough so that students initiate and actively explore them on their own. This is an ideal learning situation since it fosters independence and an opportunity for students to learn by exploration and trial and error.

Whenever students demonstrate sufficient interest and ability, this approach should be used. While this is appropriate for students at any age, it is particularly important for young children, because it teaches them that their environment is an interesting place and it encourages them to develop interests beyond their own bodies. When students are young, the instructor needs to work with their families to identify materials and adaptations that are most effective.

This type of programming can be used for students at different ability levels.   **Examples**

Young preschoolers in a play environment:

This might include setting up a high contrast glare-free background such as a light or dark mat on the floor (depending on the toys that will be used), ensuring that the toys have bold designs or clear markings so they can be seen easily, and placing the toys within the students' visual range. It may be helpful to include some toys that make sounds when touched and musical toys that wind up to make sounds. It may also be helpful to give the students visual cues about what to do with the toys such as highlighting the connectors on snap beads or the wind up key on an action toy. Once the environment has been set up to include toys that should appeal to the students' interest and ability levels, the students are encouraged to play for a period of time in this environment either alone or with others without adult intervention. Specific teaching at this time would interfere with the intended spontaneity and freedom that this setting offers. When students need specific instruction in how to interact with particular toys, this can be done at a different time within the natural context of playtime.

Elementary-aged students who are developmentally delayed who are learning to set the table:

Initial instruction may be needed to teach students what goes on the table and where items should be placed. However, there are ways to set up the environment to enhance independence in performing the task. This would include seeing that the dishes are stored at eye level and using a contrasting background to make them highly visible. Silverware can be kept in a divided tray of contrasting color as well. The table can be set with placemats or a tablecloth of contrasting color. Once students have had initial instruction in how to set the table, bold and simple visual cue cards can be used to remind them how the pieces are lined up or what additional serving items are needed. It is hoped that with this support, students can independently perform the task without supervision or verbal cueing.

Adolescent academic students setting up their desks for maximum visual efficiency:

Students might choose to use a dark blotter to create a glare-free contrasting surface for reading and writing, and a goose-necked reading lamp with a rheostat. Color coded folders or folders with large labels can be used to organize subjects and kept in a box or divider within easy reach. Low vision devices should also be kept in a designated place within easy reach.

VISUAL SKILLS TRAINING

Visual skills training is a deliberate attempt to work with students to teach specific visual attending behaviors such as fixating on or following an object. The instructor introduces the visual stimulus. One way that this may be done with a young child is by establishing eye contact, as the human face is a motivating stimulus and an important part of social/emotional development. A light, mobile or toy with bold designs could also be used. When visual attention occurs, the child is reinforced. This type of programming is primarily for students who have not been exposed to visual experiences because it was assumed that they could not see anything, or because their visual environment was not stimulating for some other reason. While research on the advantages of visual skills training is inconclusive, **the general consensus is that it is most beneficial for young children while their visual system is still in development and not very helpful for students who are developmentally delayed or for whom generalizing to different situations is difficult.** Older students and students who are multiply impaired would benefit more from the next type of training, visually dependent task training.

Another group of students who may benefit from visual skills training is those who have recently experienced cerebral trauma (e. g., anoxia, head injury, encephalitis, or meningitis). It has been noted that vision tends to improve during the first 18 months to two years after the injury (Groenveld et al, 1990). Specific programming may be helpful in facilitating this visual improvement. See pages 16 and 17 for suggestions on programming for students who have severe cortical visual impairments.

Visual skills training is most efficient when it uses real objects from the students' world. These objects may need to be adapted for high visibility. Special lighting may be used to call attention to them. While rewards for looking at the object can be unrelated (e.g., food or touch), it is more effective when the looking can activate a natural reward such as a drink from the cup that a student just looked at or turning on a musical toy once a student has looked at it.

Since this type of programming teaches "looking for the sake of looking," it is an important first step in developing functional vision. However, **students should be assisted to move from this level as quickly as possible so that they can experience success in using their vision to complete tasks.**

An example of using visual skills training includes painting black dots or **Examples**
stripes on baby' bottles and then holding it in front of the baby until he
focuses on it before giving it to him. Another example is putting bold
colored clothing with visually interesting patterns on a young child (e.g.,
bold checked or striped socks or shoes on a young baby so she can see
her feet more easily). Another possibility is playing a hide and seek game
can be played by shining a light on different objects which the students
have to find. Additional suggestions for activities can be found in *Preschool
Vision Stimulation: It's More Than A Flashlight!* (Harrell & Akeson, 1987).

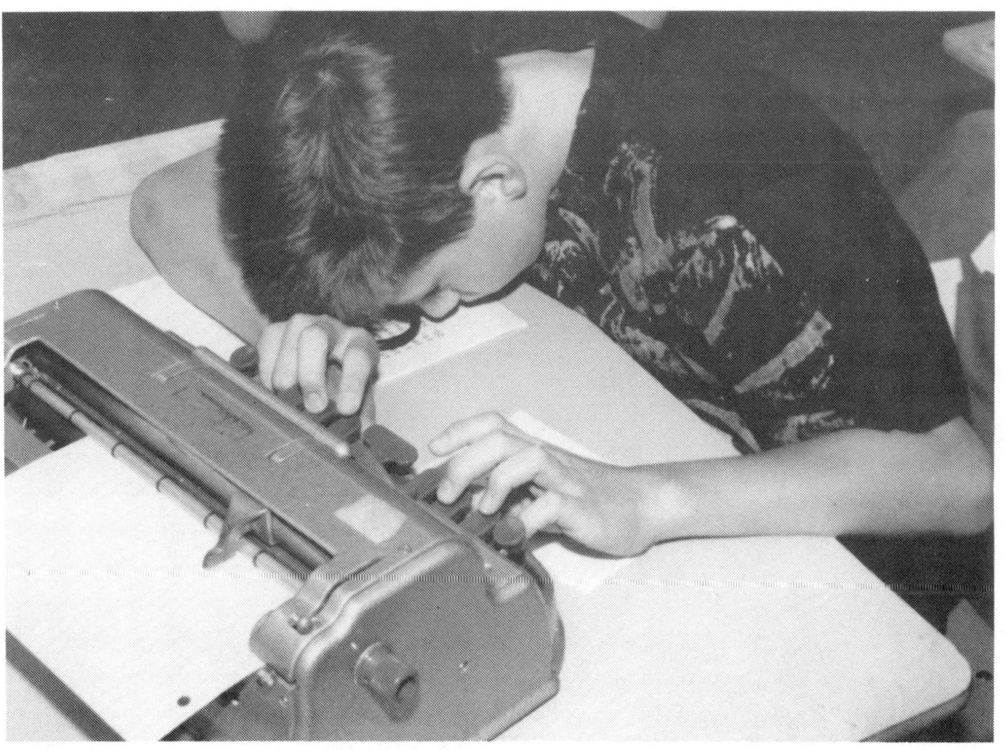

VISUALLY DEPENDENT TASK TRAINING

Visually dependent task training occurs when visual attending behaviors are applied to specific tasks in order to promote visual-cognitive and visual-motor behaviors. This teaches students to use their vision in meaningful, functional activities. The instructors introduce the activities to the students, identify the visual behavior that the students need to develop in order to complete tasks more efficiently, motivate them to perform desired visual behaviors, and reinforce students when they occur. Ideally tasks should be designed so that the actions that students produce are rewarding in themselves. When this is not possible an external reward may be needed but should be faded as quickly as possible. Visually dependent task training can be applied to activities in all aspects of students' lives wherever they can benefit from learning how to use their vision to perform tasks more efficiently.

This type of training can be very diversified. It can include teaching students how to use their vision to perform a specific task such as lining up a button and buttonhole when hanging a shirt on a hanger, or using the lessons in the *Program to Develop Efficiency in Visual Functioning* (Barraga, 1980) for specific academically oriented visual tasks. This type of programming could also include specific instruction in the use of low vision devices.

A young student with multiple impairments who is learning to drink from a cup:

This task would include expecting a student to look at the cup, recognize it, and then reach for the cup to secure the drink. The instructor might place a highly visible cup in a place where a student would be able to see it. If he does not immediately look at the cup, the teacher might cue him to do so. If he looks at the cup and does not reach for it, the teacher might physically prompt him to reach for the cup and bring it to his mouth. Students would demonstrate visual attending behaviors when they focused on the cup independently. They would demonstrate visual cognitive behaviors when they identified that it was a cup that had something to drink in it. Finally they would demonstrate visual motor skills when they reached for the cup and brought it to their mouth. In this instance the drink is its own reward. However, students may also need positive feedback about how effectively it was done.

Other examples of this type of training include:

- **An academic elementary age student who is learning how to write, or using a low vision device to read the blackboard.**

- **Adolescent students who are multiply impaired who are learning how to line up clothing when folding it, matching to sample when locating objects in a grocery store, and identifying a menu selection from a choice book in a restaurant.**

There are two principles that should dominate all considerations when planning instructional modification:

- **Help students attain the maximum use of vision with the least amount of modification.**

- **Help students develop a realistic balance between what is possible and what is practical.**

While it is generally better to expect more of students than to expect less, be alert for signs of frustration which can signal the upper limits of visual functioning. When these visual limits have been reached, problem solve alternative methods or adaptations that can ease the visual task. Use common sense and careful analysis of the task to develop practical ideas that work for particular students and do not hesitate to create original solutions to unique problems. Trial and error can be just as effective in determining effective adaptations as "textbook" recommendations.

Evaluation

It is important that the evaluation of students' visual performance be a part of the evaluation of the entire task. If a student is having difficulty learning the task, look to see if further adaptations are necessary, or whether the task is simply too difficult and cannot be adapted further. If so, break the task into even smaller steps, set up the task with a partner so that the student can partially participate, or as a last resort, discontinue that activity. If students lose interest in the task, it may be necessary to modify it to renew interest. Sometimes during attempts to modify a task, students discover a more efficient way to do it by themselves. This should always be encouraged and supported.

Barraga, N. C. & Erin, J. N. (1992). Tactual, auditory, and visual development and learning. In *Visual handicaps and learning* (3rd ed.). Austin, TX: ProEd.

Barraga, N. C. & Morris, J. E. (1980). *Program to develop efficiency in visual functioning: Source book on low vision.* Louisville, KY: American Printing House for the Blind.

Corn, A. L. (1983). Visual function: A theoretical model for individuals with low vision. *Journal of Visual Impairment and Blindness, 77,* 8, 373-377.

Corn, A. L. (1986). Low vision and visual efficiency. In G. T. Scholl (Ed.), *Foundations of education for blind and visually handicapped children and youth: Theory and practice.* New York: American Foundation for the Blind.

Corn, A. L. (1989). Instruction in the use of vision for children and adults with low vision: A proposed program model. *RE:view, 21,* 1, 26-38.

Downing, J. & Bailey, B. (1990). Developing vision use within functional daily activities for students with visual and multiple disabilities. *RE:view, 21,* 4, 209-220.

Fellows, R. R., Leguire, L. E., Rogers, G. L., & Bremer, D. L. (1986). A theoretical approach to vision stimulation. *Journal of Visual Impairment and Blindness, 80,* 8, 907-909.

Goetz, L. & Gee, K. (1987a). Functional vision programming: A model for teaching visual behaviors in natural contexts. In L. Goetz, D. Guess, & K. Stremel-Campbell (Eds.), *Innovative program design for individuals with dual sensory impairments.* Baltimore: Paul Brooks.

Goetz, L. & Gee, K. (1987b). Teaching visual attention in functional contexts: Acquisition and generalization of complex visual motor skills. *Journal of Visual Impairment and Blindness, 81,* 3,115-117.

Groenveld, M., Jan, J. E., & Leader, P. (1990). Observations on the habilitation of children with cortical visual impairment. *Journal of Visual Impairment and Blindness, 84,* 1, 11-15.

Hall, A. & Bailey, I. L. (1989). A model for training vision functioning. *Journal of Visual Impairment and Blindness, 83,* 8, 390-396.

Harrell, L. & Akeson, N. (1987). *Preschool vision stimulation: It's more than a flashlight!* New York: American Foundation for the Blind.

Hazekamp, J. & Huebner, K. M. (1989). *Program planning and evaluation for blind and students with visual impairments: National guidelines for educational excellence.* New York: American Foundation for the Blind.

Hupp, S. C. & Rosen, S. (1985). The team approach to designing instruction for visually impaired multiply handicapped children: A decision-making paradigm. *Education of the Visually Handicapped, 17,* 3, 85-96.

Mettler, R. (1990). An integrated, problem-solving approach to low vision training. *Journal of Visual Impairment and Blindness, 84,* 4, 171-177.

Smith, A. J. & Cote, K. S. (1982). *Look at me: A resource manual for the development of residual vision in multiply impaired children.* Philadelphia: Pennsylvania College of Optometry Press.

Adaptations

Adaptations of specific materials or the environment can help students who are visually impaired function more efficiently. The following section describes a variety of adaptations that might be helpful to students with visual impairments. While some specific suggestions for adaptations have been included, the list is in no way inclusive and does not imply that these adaptations would be appropriate for all students. It is essential to evaluate individual students' needs before trying any of these adaptations. Some of these adaptations are for students who have low levels of visual functioning, and some are for students who are seriously developmentally delayed. Some students may need only the mildest adaptation in one of these categories, while others may need several significant adaptations in many of the categories to perform visually.

In this chapter adaptations have been divided into the following categories:

- Adaptations in color and contrast
- Adaptations in illumination
- Adaptations in space and arrangement
- Adaptations in size and distance
- Low vision devices
- Adaptations to visual cues
- Adapting the materials
- Modifying the immediate workspace
- Modifying the larger environment

It is often effective to use bold visible colors and high contrast between colors to highlight an object which needs to be seen. The effectiveness of a particular color will vary with the visual ability of the student.

- The contrast of an object against its background is a significant factor in improving visibility (e. g., light objects on dark mats, dark objects on light counters or cutting boards, using a dark toothbrush in a white toothbrush holder, putting white shoelaces in dark sneakers).

- When choosing toys or tools for students, consider the color and contrast of the object itself (e. g., a bright yellow ball with one wide black stripe draws a child's attention better than a solid blue one).

- High contrast of letters on a page may improve visual functioning (e. g., black letters on a white background). Sometimes, white letters on a black background are easier for students to see and can reduce glare (e. g., reversed polarity on a CCTV).

- Bolder and well spaced letters are often easier to see than larger letters.

- Dark pens, markers, and soft leaded pencils may be helpful. The width and color of the line on writing paper should be selected according to the student's individual visual needs and preferences.

- A highlighting pen can be used to draw students' attention to certain words and improve contrast between the print and the page.

- Avoid using thin paper. However, if students must read something that is written on paper that is thin or poor quality, placing a sheet of dark paper under the page may help reduce "bleed through."

- The contrast of ditto-blue materials may be improved by using yellow-tinted glasses. A sheet of yellow acetate may also help to increase contrast, but it can also reduce color perception and increase glare.

The amount of light needed for individual tasks is based on individual preferences. For some students this need changes at different times of the day.

- Most frequently, evenly-distributed softly-diffused indirect lighting is recommended.

- If *reduced* illumination is needed, adjustments may need to be made such as creating shaded areas, adjusting window shades in one section of the classroom, using rheostats on overhead lights, facing away from light sources, using prescribed tinted glasses, or using prescribed pin-hole lenses or a cap with a brim.

- If *increased* illumination is needed, it may be helpful to use a small desk lamp, preferably with a rheostat control. Position the supplementary light source so that it shines directly onto the task. Ideally, the light should come from behind and over the students' shoulder. Students may need to move closer to the light source, but not so that it is directed into their eyes. Using a reading stand may increase lighting on the materials and prevent shadows. It may help to use a lighted pen or an illuminated magnification device.

- If students who have multiple disabilities are positioned on the floor for some activities, instructors should position themselves in the same place to experience what the lighting situation is and determine whether it is conducive to the students' visual performance. (Corn, 1986).

- Whenever possible surfaces within the normal viewing area of the students should be glare-free (e.g., blackboards, windows, cabinet doors, wall surfaces). Colored paper or paper with a matte finish can be used to cover surfaces. The angle of view can also be changed to reduce glare (e.g., tilting computer screens or books). Paper copies of overhead projections can be used.

- "Daylight or pink" fluorescent lighting is usually preferred to the "blue-white" type generally found in overhead fixtures. Although fluorescent lighting can generally provide higher levels of illumination, the fixtures may require increased maintenance and monitoring to eliminate flickering which sometimes comes from weak fluorescent tubes or malfunctioning starters. Incandescent lighting is usually softer but may not provide enough light when used in overhead fixtures. Even distribution and adequate diffusion are important in most cases.

- Colored lights such as flashlights or penlights with colored caps, colored Christmas-tree lights, and colored "flicker" lights can be used to get the students' visual attention. When paired with a switch and control unit, they can be used to teach cause and effect as well as visual attention. **However, if the lights have no functional applications for the students, they should be used in limited circumstances.** They should be used cautiously with students who are seizure-prone, and care should always be taken to prevent injury.

- Although ultraviolet light or "black light" has been suggested as a vision stimulation procedure, a number of research projects have suggested the need for extreme caution in its use. Children who have had cataracts removed may be at risk for retinal damage because the lens of the eye is thought to absorb ultraviolet light, which prevents it from reaching the sensitive retinal tissue. Aphakic individuals (those whose lens has been removed) do not have this possible protection from ultraviolet light. **When using ultraviolet light, protective glasses that specifically screen out ultraviolet light have been recommended for both instructors and learners** (Knowlton, 1986).

- Illumination can be used to draw attention to an object or figure by shining a light on it.

- Students should avoid looking at a light source. Not only is it uncomfortable, but it also reduces the amount of detail seen, especially through binoculars and telescopes. **Looking into a strong light source can cause retinal damage especially to students who have aphakia.**

The distance between objects, and the object's location on a page or surface affect the students' ability to see and observe detail. Inner detail and overall shape will also relate to the space and arrangement of the object.

• When it is important for students to focus on an object or person, the background should be considered. Busy environmental clutter makes it difficult to pick out the object or person. For example, a teacher may wear a splashy print with bright colors and a contrasting pattern in order to help students track her movements. However, if the teacher held an object in front of the splashy print, students may have difficulty seeing the object against that background. Consequently, the object may have to be moved away from the print or a simple contrasting background would need to be held behind the object.

• It may be helpful to reduce the number of choices or items that students are asked to look at.

• Limiting the visual clutter of the object itself may help (e.g., simplifying patterns, using solid colors with high contrast, reducing extraneous details).

• It may be necessary to reduce the information on a page. Problems or sentences can be arranged in such a way that they have "white space" between and/or around them. Parts of a page can be covered (e.g., covering the part of the page that has not been read and revealing each new line as the students move down the page, isolating words or phrases, "whiting out" extraneous information, using a typoscope or template).

Visual efficiency can be improved by increasing or decreasing the size of the objects being viewed. This can be done by using devices for magnification and minification or by varying the distance between the viewer and the original.

• There are four different kinds of magnification (Brilliant, 1983):

  1. Angular magnification causes an image to appear larger than it actually is when looking through an optical device. The magnification is produced by the optical aid not by changing the object which is being viewed.
  2. Relative distance magnification occurs when the distance is reduced between the eye and the object to be seen. High plus lenses called microscopes bring the object closer to the eye which spreads the image so as to allow it to fall on a larger area of retina. The brain is then able to read the image more easily. This strategy does not actually magnify the object.
  3. Relative size magnification increases the size of the object and generally does not require the use of an optical aid. Large print or a larger television screen are examples.
  4. Projection magnification involves projecting an image on a screen where it can be magnified. Slide projectors and closed circuit televisions are examples of projection magnification.

• The optimal position or location of students must be considered. Some examples include students who may need to use a low vision device or walk up to view something more closely and students with vision in the left eye who may need to sit on the right side of the classroom. If students have restricted fields but good acuity, they may prefer to move back to see the whole figure. However, when a change is made to the distance, other factors such as glare and lighting patterns must be considered as they may affect the students' visual abilities.

• Since being close to an object can result in automatic magnification, students may lean closer to an object or bring an object near their eyes.

- The working environment may need to be arranged to ensure comfortable posture for students. Sample adaptations might include adjusting the height of desks, tables, and chairs. Also, reading stands with moving shelves can be used, or books can be placed under the book being read to raise it up to a comfortable position.

- Reading materials can be enlarged using a copier, and large print books can be used. There are several disadvantages to large print books including the limitations in availability, the fact that they are often poorly reproduced with poor contrast, and illustrations are usually difficult to see. Also their bulky size sets students apart from their peers. For these reasons, adapting all reading materials into large print is not recommended unless it is for a temporary period until the student can be evaluated for potential use of low vision devices and the necessary instruction can be provided with these devices. **If a student cannot attain a functional reading speed using low vision devices to read regular size print, then braille should be introduced as a complimentary tool for literacy.** However, it may be functional for the student to have occasional print materials enlarged for a specific purpose. If print is to be enlarged, experiment with type sizes to see which is most preferable. Copy machines that enlarge can be set at 129% to produce 16 pt. type. Enlargement of 155% will produce 18 pt. type.

- With practice and training, some students may learn to use smaller print.

9 pt.:   Normal type size in adult books (1.5mm lower case height)

10 pt.:   Normal type size in adult books (2mm)

12 pt.:   Normal type size in children's books (2.5mm)

14 pt.:   Normal type size in children's books (3mm)

16 pt.:   12 pt. photocopied at 129% (3.5mm)

18 pt.:   12 pt. photocopied at 155% (3.5mm)

18 pt.:   Large type books (4mm)

24 pt.:   Large type books (5mm)

Low vision devices are tools that students who are visually impaired can use to see objects at a distance, read regular print, or do close work. They can be divided into optical devices and non-optical devices. Many of them will be described below. Many of these devices require instruction and practice to use efficiently, some are very delicate and require extreme care, and some are very expensive. In spite of these challenges, they can often provide the ideal adaptation because they can be used for a variety of visual tasks giving students much freedom and flexibility. Instead of adapting each task or situation, students can use one adaptation for many tasks.

Some students are reluctant to use low vision devices because they call attention to their impairment and single them out as different from their peers. Often, students will change this resistance as they discover how much they can see with the device, as their self-esteem and acceptance of their visual impairment grows, and as they experience acceptance from their peers when they use a low vision device.

It may be necessary to include instruction in use of low vision devices on the student's IEP. Specific skills in the use and care of adapted devices, including low vision devices, can be found in the goal on Self-advocacy in *Independent Living: A Curriculum with Adaptations for Students with Visual Impairments* (Loumiet & Levack, 1991, pp. 199-212).

Lenses which are placed between the eye and the object being viewed are called optical devices. Many of these devices require careful orientation and training in order to produce successful experiences. Techniques for training can be found in Chapter 12 "Distance Training Techniques" and Chapter 13 "Near Training Techniques" in *Understanding Low Vision* (Jose, 1983).

• *Hand-held magnifiers* give users the ability to adjust the working distance. They can be used in a variety of situations, are small, are inexpensive, can fit in a pocket or purse and are often more socially acceptable since they are familiar to most people. They are less effective when high power is needed and when both hands are needed for a task. They also require good eye-hand coordination. More than one power of magnification can be carried in the same case and lenses can be combined to create a third power.

Magnifiers

• *Stand mounted magnifiers* can be placed directly on the page and provide a fixed distance between lens and object. Some have good light-gathering capacity and can be equipped with additional illumination and/or additional lenses. Some can be focused. Although these magnifiers are helpful for students who have tremors or do not have good eye-hand coordination, they can cause physical discomfort if students have to lean close to the lens for long periods of time and they are less convenient to carry. Goosenecked magnifiers allow students to adjust the lens and then use both hands for working, but have low magnification power.

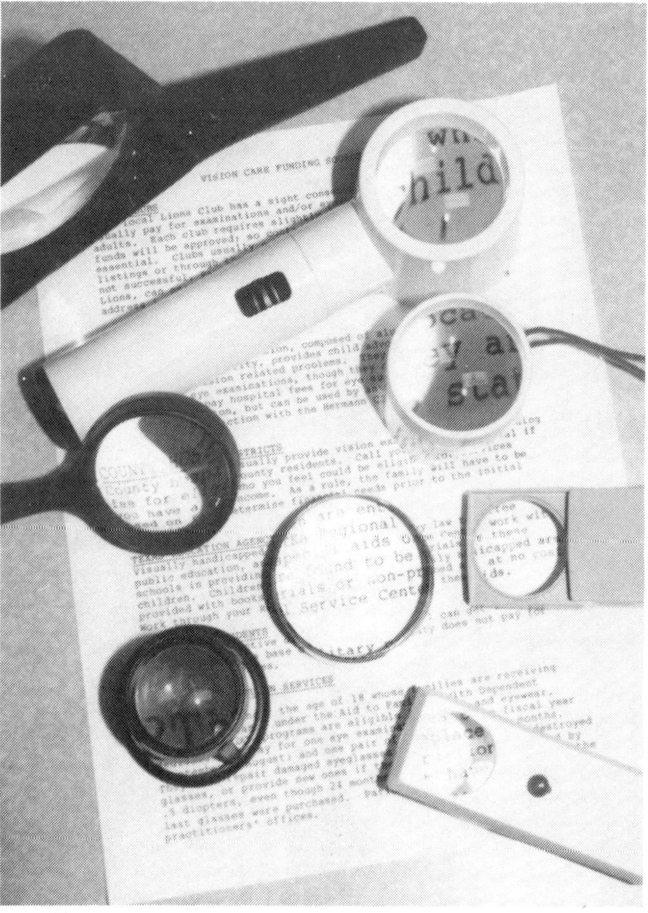

Telescopes These are designed for distance viewing. Most of them can be focused. Afocal telescopes are focused for infinity and are not adjustable to intermediate distances. Types of telescopes include:

- *Hand-held monoculars* can be used for observing or tracking objects at a distance. The viewer brings it to the eye for the widest field of view. Depending on the students' visual abilities and preferences, they can be used with either hand or eye and with other prescription lenses (though placing them in front of a lens will reduce the visual field). They do restrict the use of one hand and can cause arm fatigue if used for a long period of time. Using a hand-held magnifier does require some instruction to learn how to align the object, the lens and eye; how to scan for objects; how to follow a moving object; and how to hold the aid steadily. They are especially helpful for viewing the chalkboard, for seeing theater and sporting events, and for seeing street signs or reading the numbers on a bus. Another advantage of hand-held monoculars is their small size. They can easily be kept in a pocket or purse or hung around the neck.

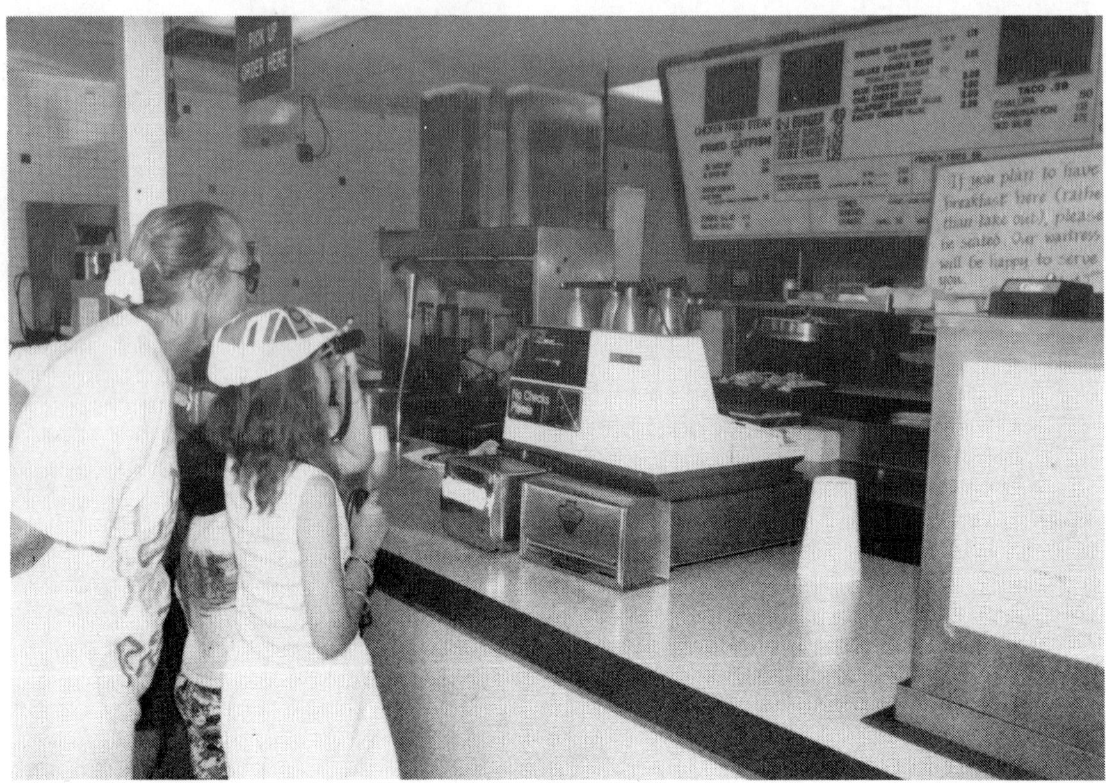

- *Spectacle mounted monoculars* free the students' hands to perform tasks. They can be used when shopping and in general mobility. In some states, including Texas, they can be used for driving if the person is trained and meets other specific criteria for a driver's license.

- *Binoculars* can be used for short term distance viewing when students have vision in both eyes and can fuse an image. They can provide a larger field and make it easier to find targets, but are larger and heavier than monoculars and much more conspicuous.

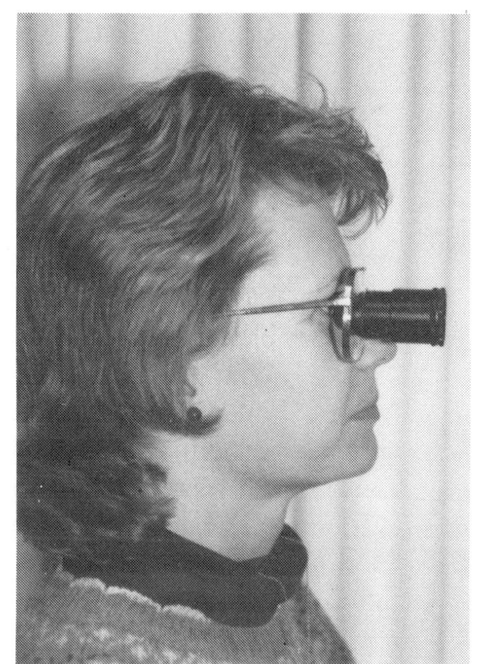

- *Clip-on telescopes* can be put on glasses as needed. A telescope can be clipped on either or both lenses for long term distance viewing or when students need to use both hands. The lens on a telescope is farther from the eye which reduces the visual field. Some are mounted off center and above the pupil, but when the telescope covers the eye, students cannot move around when it is used.

- *Full-field telescopes* cover the entire lens and must be used when students are stationary. They are prescribed for specific vocational and recreational needs.

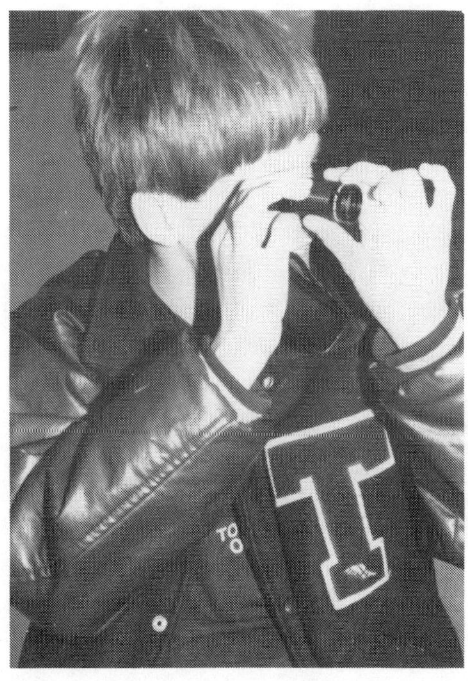

- *Bioptic telescopes* are mounted right into the lenses. Since these miniaturized telescopes do not cover the entire lens, students can move around. By lowering the head and raising the eyes they can look through the telescope for distance viewing. When looking straight through the conventional lens, the students do not have restricted peripheral view. The telescope can be mounted in one or both lenses and more than one correction can be put in the lens. These lenses are more costly and fragile. They require training and practice in head and eye positioning for various viewing needs. Cosmetically, they may cause some problems; however, behind the lens bioptic lenses are now available and these are less noticeable since they do not protrude from the front of the lens. Also, since extra head movements are needed to function with bioptics (beyond those required with hand held monoculars), they may not be the mounting system of choice for students who do not want to be moving their heads in order to view notes on the chalkboard. In some states, including Texas, they can be used for driving with specific training for those who qualify.

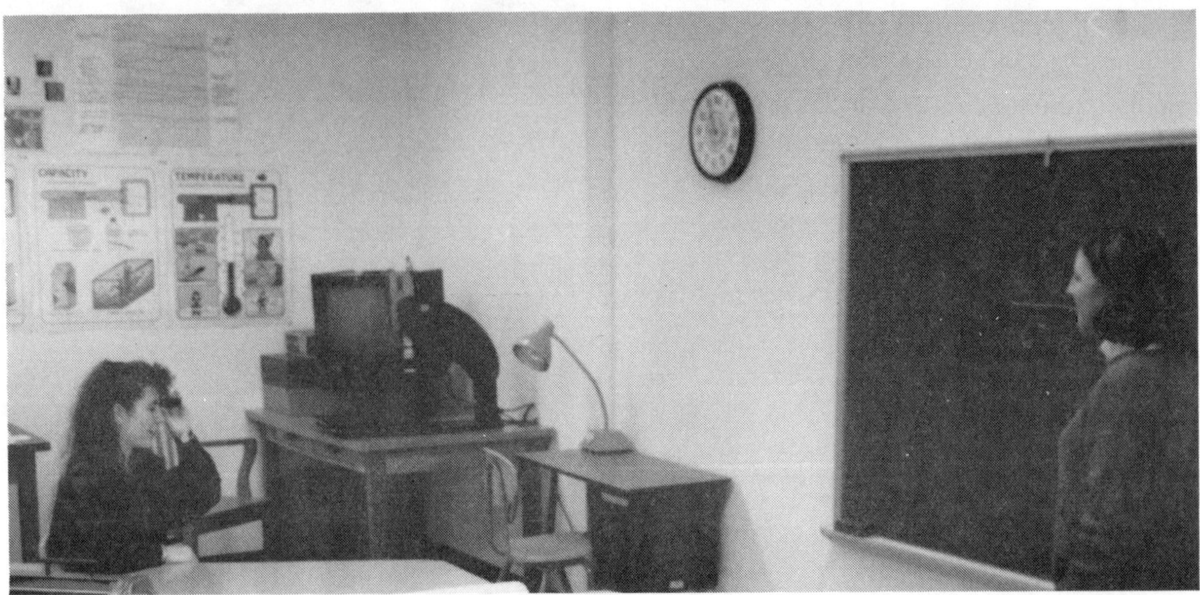

- *Telemicroscopes* (also known as reading telescopes or surgical telescopes) are distance telescopes which have been modified to allow a fixed working distance that is closer to the normal working distance. If a reading cap has been affixed to the telescope, it can be removed for distance viewing and then added for the specific task. Different caps can be put on for different needs. Telemicroscopes do have a smaller field of view than a regular microscope. They have depth perception changes because of vertical displacement which means that students must lower their heads more to find a target. Movement is often exaggerated in higher powered models.

Microscopes

Microscopes are plus lenses that bring the object closer to the eye which spreads the image to allow it to fall on a larger area of the retina. They can be head borne or frame mounted. When they are designed for near viewing they are called "reading telescopes". Increased magnification results in shorter working distance which can cause fatigue. Distance acuity is blurred when using them.

Field Utilization Aids

Visually impaired people who have tunnel vision will be assisted by minifying telescopes or reverse telescopes, field expanders such as prisms and mirrors for peripheral awareness, minus lenses, and scanning training.

- *Reverse telescopes* or minus lenses minify objects at a distance thereby increasing the field of view. The disadvantage is that since the objects are smaller, detail is lost. They may facilitate travel for people with restricted peripheral vision, known as tunnel vision, if they have good central vision and skills in scanning and tracking.

- *Prisms* "bring in" peripheral vision through the use of small prism lenses that are placed on the edge of the central viewing area of the prescription lens. Students can then glance into the prism that displaces the object from the periphery to the central viewing area where it can be seen. They create additional cognitive processing problems due to distortion of the visual field and take time, effort, and training to use effectively.

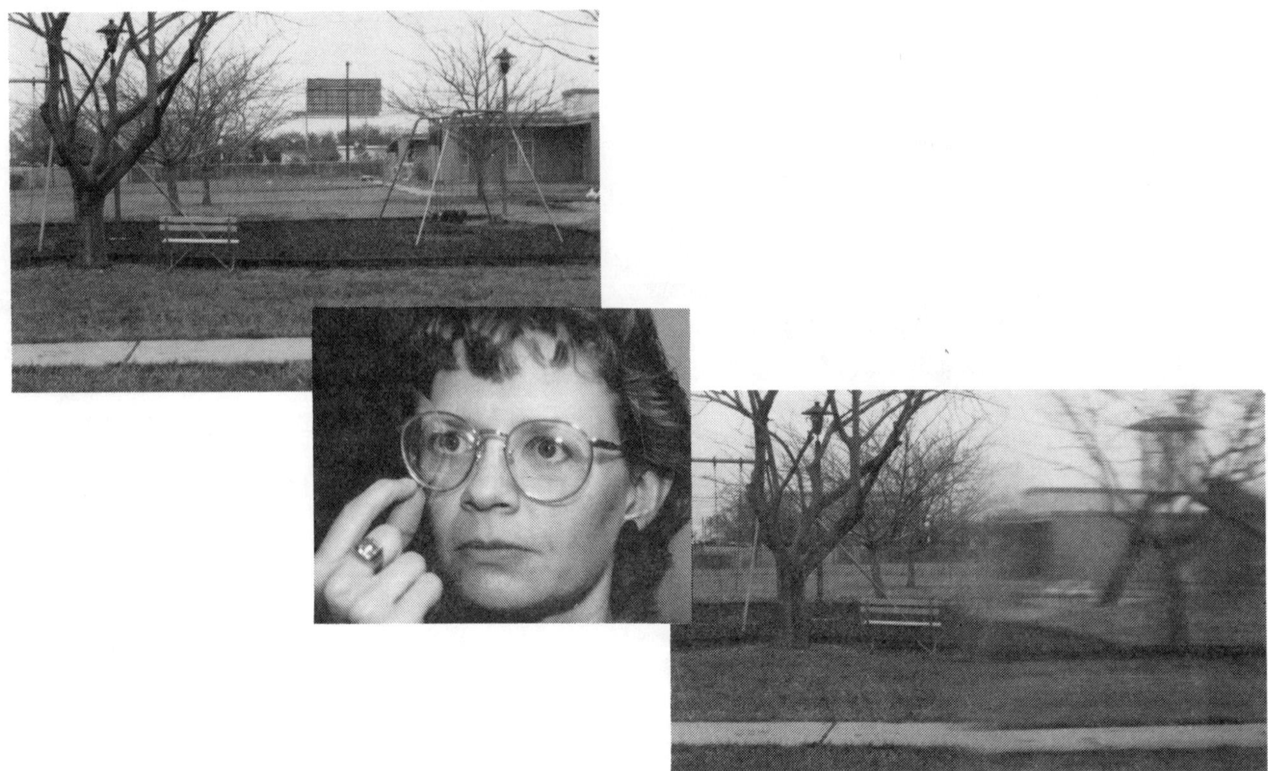

- *Contact lenses* are effective especially with refractive errors of +10 or -10 diopters. They provide more light, wider field, and fewer distortions than regular lenses. If a student has a small visual field, they are more effective than thick glasses which limit functional fields. They are also lighter than glasses with thick lenses. Contact lenses are particularly helpful for students who have corneal distortions. Since the telescope can be brought very close to the eye for a larger field, their use with contact lenses makes an effective combination. For some students a telescope can be devised with up to 2X magnification using a high powered contact lens and an aphakic or cataract lens.

- *Night-vision scope* is a light intensification unit that provides enough light to the retina in dark situations so that the central vision is stimulated. It is used like a monocular telescope by students with night blindness. It helps students function in outdoor settings at night or in low levels of illumination, but is not widely used.

Other Optical Devices

NON-OPTICAL DEVICES

Machines which electronically enlarge an image are called electronic magnifiers. While this method can be helpful for specific needs, it is not recommended as a general adaptation for all printed material. These electronic magnifiers can be used in conjunction with optical devices to provide a full range of adaptations for students who have low vision. They are used to read regular size print is often preferable to large print production, since it allows the reader more flexibility and accessibility. It is important to note, however, that all visual impairments are not enhanced by the use of magnification or enlargement.

Closed Circuit Televisions (CCTV's)

A CCTV (Closed Circuit Television) provides electronic magnification. A video camera is used to capture blocks of text or images which are then enlarged either electronically or through a lens and displayed on a monitor. Most CCTV's made in 1989 or later use a CCD (Charged Coupled Device) camera. Features of these units include: enhanced contrast, brightness and clarity of images, less "ghosting" of letters when text is moved, increased depth of field, and no "'burn-in" of images left under the camera for extended time.

The majority of current CCTV's are **"in-line"** systems. The monitor, camera and electronics are all arranged in a single vertical line above the reading material (placed on a reading tray known as an X/Y table which moves vertically and horizontally on a fixed frame). Monitor sizes vary from 12" to 19" (19"+ Monitors are generally placed side-by-side to the camera). Most units include a height adjustment, however it is generally recommended that the system be placed on a lower than normal table or desk, to allow the student to view the monitor at a comfortable eye level. Larger monitors often increase reading speed, because more words can appear on a larger screen without altering print size.

In-line CCTV's magnifications vary ranging between 5X-60X. As noted in previous sections, using high magnification, provides fewer words on the screen, slowing the reading pace. Students should be encouraged to utilize the smallest amount of magnification necessary to comfortably function and perform tasks.

Common CCTV features include:
- X/Y table margin stops: for example, when print columns need to be read, the stops will hold the table at a position where only one columns will be viewed at a time
- X/Y table drag control: loosens or tightens the movement of the table (e. g., tighten if motor control is poor)
- focus, contrast and enlargement controls: adjust to individual needs
- windowing: parts of the text can be blocked to allow single line viewing for example
- positive and negative polarity: white on black or black on white

CCTV options include:
- computer access systems where the monitor can show computer information as well as magnification of printed materials
- external cameras for long distance (blackboard) or short focus (typewriter)
- motorized X/Y tables
- amber or green monitors (acetate filters can also be utilized on standard black/white monitors)

Color CCTV's can offer students access to photographs, maps, color-coded charts and information not readily identified by black and white systems. However, where sighted people are often fascinated by color, many people with low vision cannot see colors adequately. Color systems tend to reduce contrast and clarity, making general reading tasks difficult and tedious.

Portable and Handscan CCTV's are becoming more popular, both as the technology improves and as students may have access to them as a secondary system. A portable CCTV may have a 4"-14" screen, with a hand-held camera attached to electronics which may be carried in a case or briefcase. When portability is absolutely necessary, the 4" monitors may be helpful, however, connection to a TV or other monitor may be suitable for other tasks. Some notable advantages to handscan cameras, include their ability to easily point to the image to be enlarged, simplifying the X/Y table search. Often focusing is not necessary because they have a "fixed focus". Handwriting with a portable unit is usually possible with a separate handwriting adapter. These units can be as costly as "in-line" systems, and the student's responsibility for the equipment should be considered.

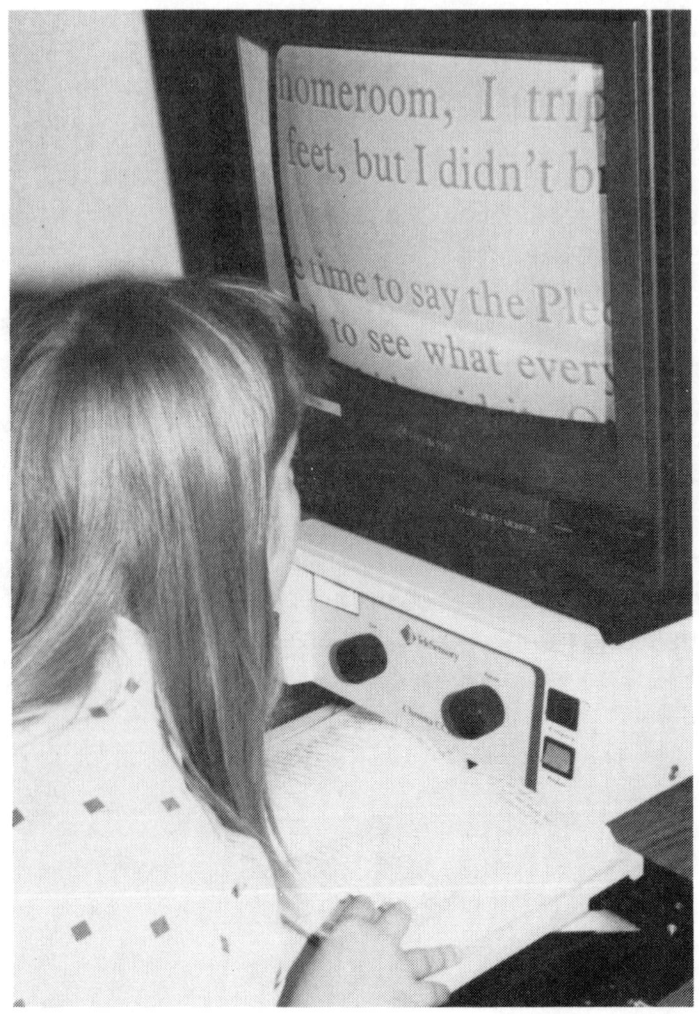

Magnified Visual Output:

Large Print (and/or graphics) on a computer screen is available for low vision students. This can be done on most Apple, IBM compatible, or Macintosh format computers. Some large print access is performed by software only, while others use both hardware and software. Some operate from the keyboard, others may use a mouse or joystick. Some programs can produce large print on a printer. A color monitor can provide a variety of background and foreground colors for enhancing text and graphics. No one program best meets all students needs. Consider magnification choices, available fonts, student preferences. Computer information needed to determine which system may best meet your students needs include the type of computer, amount of memory, names and type of software you wish to run (text or graphics), and computers graphics capability. Demonstration software is often available for these types of programs.

Electronic Voice Output:

Speech Output from a computer can be utilized by low vision students. This can be in conjunction with, or instead of large print access. For some students, especially those requiring a lot of magnification, enlarged print on the computers' screen proves slow and tedious. Speech can be a faster, less tiresome way to use a computer. Viewing distance, reading speed, as well as a student's attention span should be considered in determining the use of large print and/or speech. Speech output on a computer consists of two components - a speech synthesizer and screen-reading software. When considering using both large print and speech together, be careful that both programs are compatible.

Electronic Input Devices:

Optical Character Recognition Systems **(Scanners)** are available for scanning print information into a computer. Once the information is "scanned" into a computer, a low vision student can access that information via large print output on a monitor or from an inkprint printer, electronic speech output, and braille output. Some scanners attach to a standard computer, while others are stand alone units with speech output. These units can often be found within a regional center or library, and are often used by individuals who are learning disabled or persons who are visually impaired.

Evaluating for Technology Needs

When making decisions about technology, the following questions may be helpful.

- What are the student's physical or mental strengths and limitations?
- What are the student's needs and potential uses for electronic low vision devices?
- What other low vision devices is the student currently using, if any?
- What other current technology is used or has been used by the student?
- What is the increased learning potential?
- Will the student be motivated to use an electronic low vision device?
- Can the student be responsible in handling an electronic low vision device?
- What goals for the future does the student have?
- What are the best modes of output needed as determined in the *Functional Low Vision Assessment?*
- Who will train the student in the use of the device?
- Who will monitor the student in the use of the device?
- Who pays for the purchase of an electronic low vision device?
- What electronic equipment is offered by the school or social services?
- When will the device be needed?

- *Photocopy enlarging* should depend on the abilities, ages, and preferences of students. Large print should be the last choice when enlargement is effective, since it restricts the reader to only enlarged texts and takes time and money to produce.

- *Photography* and *video cameras* allow distant images to be zoomed in for close-up examination. While traveling, for example, students may want to capture scenes on film or videotape.

- *Projectors* can magnify an image as it is projected on a screen by adjusting the distance between the projector and the screen.

- *Wide angle mobility light* (WAML) is a headlamp that can be strapped around the waist. It gives a wide bright beam of light for students who must rely on their central vision because of deficiencies in their peripheral vision. It is helpful when students must travel at night or in low levels of illumination.

- Information about illumination control aids (e. g., lamps, dimmer switches, rheostats) can be found on pages 72 and 73.

- Information about contrast aids (e. g., typoscopes, yellow acetate, bold line paper) can be found on page 71.

- Other low vision devices such as reading and typing stands, pin-holes, large print, visors, sunshades, typoscopes, and signature and writing guides are discussed in the other sections of adaptations.

Other Nonoptical Devices

This is an important area for consideration. Frequently, modifying the visual characteristics or some of the parts of a task can make it easier to complete the task. Hall and Bailey (1989) identify three different types of cue control which the instructor can use to regulate the visual stimuli presented to students:

- **Visual conspicuity enhancement** uses color, contrast, illumination, space, arrangement, size and/or distance to make the object more visible and ensure that students can see it more easily.

- **Visual conspicuity reduction** modifies the object or environment to reduce its visual characteristics to make a task more challenging. An instructor may choose to enhance the conspicuity of an object or task at first. However, once the students are familiar with the task, the conspicuity may need to be reduced to challenge them to perform more difficult visual tasks and to use materials with the least amount of adaptation necessary. For example, after a student has learned how to pour coffee into a white cup, cups of different color could be introduced. Another example of this process could be used when teaching a student to tie a bow. Start with bright shoelaces of a contrasting color and move to less conspicuous ones.

- **Visual coding** is another option when planning instruction. It not only calls attention to the object or task but gives information about how it is to be done. An example is teaching students how to set the table by using laminated placemats that have the outline of the plate cup and spoon drawn on them. The students are expected to match the real object to the outline. Obviously, visual coding is only of use when the students can make judgements from the visual information received. Another example of visual coding is using colored or printed notebooks to code each subject during the school day for easy storage and retrieval of papers and materials.

When adaptations are needed, decisions will need to be made on whether to adapt the materials, the students' immediate work space, the larger environment, any combination of these, or all of them.

The instructor and students will need to decide about what kinds of adaptations they need for their classroom materials, particularly when they are in regular education classes. The least restrictive option is always to use commercial materials as they are, and to use low vision devices as needed. However, at times, further modification may be needed. Sometimes it is simpler and more economical to adapt available commercial materials, while other times it may be necessary to buy materials that have been specifically adapted for people with visual impairments, when these are available. It may also be necessary to purchase these adapted materials and then modify them further to meet the individual needs of the student, particularly for students who have multiple impairments.

Materials can be modified in many ways. While a few examples have been given below, the possibilities are limited only to the imagination of the instructor and the students.

- **Modifying color and contrast:**
  Use materials that contrast to their background. When the materials are not visible enough, use contrasting tape or dark markers to put lines or designs on them for higher visibility.

- **Modifying illumination:**
  Shine a light on the object to call students' attention to it.

- **Modifying space and arrangement:**
  Reduce the number of choices or items to look at on a page or choice board, or reduce the complexity of figure-ground.

- **Modifying size and distance:**
  It may be necessary to enlarge some details of materials or bring the materials closer to the students, or to the left or right, or move them further away.

Modifying the Immediate Workspace

The immediate work space means the area that the students are using while performing a task. It could be a desk, a place setting during mealtimes, the bathtub, or a counter where a cooking activity is taking place. Some general suggestions include:

- **Modifying color and contrast:**
  Items can be seen more clearly when they are against a solid, glare-free background of a contrasting color.

- **Modifying illumination:**
  Use a small desk lamp, preferably with a rheostat control; and direct the light on the materials, if increased illumination is needed.

- **Modifying space and arrangement:**
  Help the students organize materials so that they can be retrieved easily. Simplify the environment so that students have clear figure-ground distinctions.

- **Modifying size and distance:**
  Ensure that the chair and table are appropriate heights so students can work comfortably, particularly if they need to get close to their work to see it. If students need more adaptive positioning, be sure that they are physically comfortable and the materials are within their visual range.

Finally, there are times when the larger environment will need adaptation. It could include modifying a classroom, adapting a route, and organizing a home environment such as a kitchen, bedroom, or closet. While this gets more difficult when students are in mainstreamed settings, often the modifications to the environment which are helpful to students who are visually impaired are also helpful to other students. For example reducing glare can reduce eyestrain for all students. Sometimes the classroom teacher is more receptive to changing the environment when the benefit to all the students can be pointed out. Examples of how the larger environment can be modified include:

- **Modifying color and contrast:**
  Use contrasting rugs to define certain areas of a room, or place a contrasting color on pieces of furniture to make them easily identifiable, as well as on the corners of furniture to avoid bumping into them.

- **Modifying illumination:**
  Create shaded areas. Adjust window shades in one section of the classroom; use rheostats on overhead lights. Be sure that students face away from light sources. For students who have multiple disabilities, it may be helpful to reduce room illumination and then shine a light on the object that they need to look at.

- **Modifying space and arrangement:**
  Arrange furniture so that it is in a logical pattern with clear passageways. Keep furniture in consistent places. Remove low, small, or difficult to see pieces of furniture from walkways. Reduce clutter.

- **Modifying size and distance:**
  Be sure that the student's work place is at the appropriate distance (e.g., close to the instructor if distance vision is affected, farther back or to the appropriate side, if peripheral field loss occurs).

- When making decisions about adaptations, three areas must be considered. They include the **student's visual abilities** (acuity, visual fields, motility, brain functions, light and color reception), the **stored and available individuality of the student** (cognition, sensory developmental integration, perception, psychological makeup, physical makeup), and **environmental cues** (color, contrast, time, space, illumination) (Corn, 1983).

- Weigh the **extent that the adaptation calls attention to the students** and limits their performance of the task when the adaptation is not available, **against the independence that they experience** when using the adaptation.

- Develop a **realistic balance between what is possible and what is practical.** Compromises may need to be made.

- Sometimes it is most efficient to use a **combination of environmental adaptations** (e.g., adjusting lighting, highlighting or marking objects to be seen) **and personal accommodation** on the part of the student (e.g., moving closer, using a low vision device, wearing a visor to shade eyes from glare).

- Use **common sense and careful analysis** of the task to develop practical ideas that work for a particular learner.

- When possible, **help the students to identify their own visual limitations** while **encouraging maximum visual efficiency** by problem solving what kinds of adaptations might help.

- Do not hesitate to **create original solutions to unique problems.** Trial and error can be just as effective in determining effective adaptations as "textbook" recommendations.

- Generally, it is **better to expect more than to expect less.** Higher but realistic expectations tend to encourage greater effort.

- **Be alert for signs of frustration and fatigue** which can signal the upper limits of visual functioning.

- When these visual limits have been reached, **problem solve alternative methods or adaptations** that can ease the visual task.

Stratton (1990) discusses a hierarchy of least restrictive materials that should be considered when making decisions about adaptations. When this hierarchy is applied, teachers look at the students' abilities and the activity or skill that they need to learn and determine what is the minimal amount of intervention or accommodation needed to perform it independently.

In order to insure that students have the opportunity to experience as much independence as possible, it is essential to consider continually whether the adaptations are the least restrictive ones necessary to perform the task. There are four levels of adaptation:

1. At the least restrictive level, students are able to **learn from the natural environment** with no intervention or adaptation. While this is always the ideal, frequently students who are visually impaired need more intervention in order to learn.

2. The second level includes **direct intervention on the part of instructors** by either calling attention to an object or giving verbal description or physical prompting to help students understand how to perform a specific task. Again at this level the materials are not adjusted in any way.

3. The third level is **short term adaptations to materials, work spaces and the larger environment.** These adaptations make it possible for students to learn how to use the material or perform the skill. These adaptations should be a means toward independent use without adaptations. An example of this would be putting large print numbers on a telephone until students can memorize their location or learn how to use a low vision device to read them. Also, adaptations which are readily available and are not necessarily intended for students who are visually impaired would be included in this category such as felt tip pens or high-contrast, bold-faced fashion watches.

4. Finally, the highest level of adaptation requires **materials which have been specifically designed to accommodate for students' disability** and are necessary for them to perform the task. Braille, communication boards, large print timers, or low vision devices would be included in this category.

Adaptations for Students Who Also Have Cognitive Impairments

This issue becomes more complicated with students who also have cognitive impairments. Often through the use of adaptations they are capable of performing a task that would not otherwise be possible. Since many do not generalize, and since many are often unable to recognize or communicate what adaptation they are using, it is imperative that all of the people who work with these students be informed about their adaptations and have access to them. Ideally the adaptations should be documented in the lesson plans or the students' folders. When planning adaptations it is also important to think about whether this adaptation is going to be available in different settings later on in their lives. If the adaptation is necessary for students' independent performance of a functional skill, it is important that the adaptation be economical and readily available.

Once students have been identified as having learning disabilities as well as visual impairments, several adaptations can be made. These may include adaptations to the materials, adaptations to the method or approach to instruction, or adapting the immediate work space. Some of these adaptations are simply good teaching practice and would be applicable for any students. Many of these suggestions have come from Harley, Truan, & Sanford (1987).

- Be sure that the reading medium is the most effective and efficient one for the task.

- At the beginning of an assignment, review, highlight and/or write out the steps that would be needed to complete the task.

- Use linemarkers, templates or typoscopes to block out extraneous information to facilitate focusing on the task.

- Keep coded notebooks for each subject so students can organize all papers and materials according to subject.

- If students have experienced failure with one kind of material, try new materials that look different to encourage success.

- Keep print style and format simple.

**ADAPTATIONS TO
THE MATERIALS**

ADAPTATIONS TO THE METHOD OR APPROACH TO INSTRUCTION

- Use a multisensory approach which includes visual, auditory and tactual learning whenever possible.

- When students have difficulty with memory, introduce new information slowly and provide a lot of repetition.

- If students have experienced a great deal of failure, begin lessons at a level lower that their ability level to build confidence and self-esteem before approaching new and challenging work.

- Break the tasks into small, meaningful components, and teach only a few steps at a time.

- Provide extra time for students to complete their work.

- Emphasize content that reflects the students' interest and ability levels.

- Teach students to write down homework assignments and include a list of all the materials they might need to complete the assignment. These can be reviewed by an adult.

- Help students to see how each subject interrelates and supports what they are learning in other areas.

- Emphasize using a consistent approach to tasks, using a left-to-right approach whenever possible.

- Keep a consistent daily schedule, whenever possible so the students experience predictability and consistency.

- Build in extra "stress free" or relaxation activities.

- Students who have difficulty with handwriting may begin typing or word processing at an early age.

- Offer alternative methods of testing.

ADAPTATIONS TO THE IMMEDIATE WORK SPACE

- Create a study carrel where visual and auditory distractors can be reduced to encourage concentration.

- Organize materials and insist that students return them to their appropriate places.

Barraga, N. C. & Erin, J. N. (1992). Curricular adaptations and media. In *Visual handicaps and learning* (3rd ed.). Austin, TX: ProEd.

Brilliant, R. (1983). Magnification in low vision devices made simple. *Journal of Visual Impairment and Blindness, 77,* 4, 169-171.

Corn, A. L. (1980a). Functional environmental cues for the low vision individual. Excerpt from the *Interdisciplinary approach to low vision rehabilitation.* Prepared for the National Training Workshop in Low Vision, Chicago, August 25-27, 1980.

Corn, A. L. (1980b). Optical aids in the classroom. *Education of the Visually Handicapped, 12,* 4,114-119.

Corn, A. L. (1983). Visual function: A theoretical model for individuals with low vision. *Journal of Visual Impairment and Blindness, 77,* 8, 373-377.

Corn, A. L. (1985). Strategies for the enhancement of visual functioning in individuals with fixed visual deficits: An interdisciplinary model. *Rehabilitation Literature, 46,* 1-2, 8-11.

Corn, A. L. (1986). Low vision and visual efficiency. In G. T. Scholl (Ed.), *Foundations of education for blind and visually handicapped children an youth: Theory and practice.* New York: American Foundation for the Blind.

Corn, A. L. (1991). Least restrictive access to the visual environment. *Journal of Visual Impairment and Blindness, 85,* 195-197.

Corn, A. L. & Ryser, G. (1989). Access to print students with low vision. *Journal of Visual Impairment and Blindness, 83,* 340-349.

Cowan, C. & Sheplar, R. (1990). Teaching techniques for teaching young children to use low vision devices. *Journal of Visual Impairment and Blindness, 84,* 9, 419-421.

De Witt, J. C., Schreier, E. M., & Leventhal, J. D. (1988a). A look at closed circuit television systems (CCTV) for persons with low vision. *Journal of Visual Impairment and Blindness, 82,* 4, 151-160.

De Witt, J. C., Schreier, E. M., Leventhal, J. D., & Meyers, A. M. (1988b). A guide to selecting large print/enhanced image computer access hardware/software for persons with low vision. *Journal of Visual Impairment and Blindness, 82,* 10, 432-442.

Dickman, I. R. (1983). *Making life more livable: Simple adaptations for the homes of blind and visually impaired older adults.* New York: American Foundation for the Blind.

Directory of living aids for the handicapped. (1984). Santa Monica, CA: Ready Reference Press.

Efron, M., Miller-Wood, D. J., & Wood, T. A. (1989). Visual skill development for the functionally blind via closed circuit television. *Journal of Vision Rehabilitation, 3,* 4,11-16.

Faye, E. E. (Ed.). (1984). Guide to selecting reading spectacles, hand magnifiers, telescopes, electronic aids, and absorptive lenses. In *Clinical low vision* (2nd ed.). Boston: Little, Brown.

Hall, A. & Bailey, I. L. (1989). A model for training vision functioning. *Journal of Visual Impairment and Blindness, 83,* 8, 390-396.

Harley, R. K., Truan, M. B., & Sanford, L. D. (1987). Teaching techniques for visually impaired students with learning problems. In *Communication skills for visually impaired learners.* Springfield, IL: Charles Thomas.

Jackson, R. M. (1983a), Early educational use of optical aids: A cautionary note. *Education of the Visually Handicapped, 15,* 1, 20-29.

Jose, R. T. (Ed.). (1983). Treatment options. In *Understanding low vision.* New York: American Foundation for the Blind.

Jose, R. T., Spitzberg, L. A., & Kuether, C. L. (1989). A behind the lens reversed (BTLR) telescope. *Journal of Vision Rehabilitation, 3,* 2, 37-46.

Kelleher, D. K. (1979). Orientation to low vision devices. *Journal of Visual Impairment and Blindness, 73,* 5, 161-166.

Kelleher, D. K. (1982). Orientation to low vision devices. In S. Mangold (Ed.), *A teacher's guide to the special educational needs of blind and visually handicapped children.* New York: American Foundation for the Blind.

Knowlton, M. (1986). Ultraviolet light: Some considerations for vision stimulation. *Education of the Visually Handicapped, 17,* 4, 147-153.

Koenig, A. J. & Holbrook, M. C. (1989). Determining the reading medium for students with visual impairments: A diagnostic teaching approach. *Journal of Visual Impairment and Blindness, 83,* 5, 296-302.

Koenig, A. J. & Holbrook, M. C. (1991). Determining the reading medium for students with visual impairments via diagnostic teaching. *Journal of Visual Impairment and Blindness, 85,* 61-68.

Lang, M. A. & Sullivan, C. (1986). Adapting home environments for visually impaired and blind children. *Children's Environments Quarterly, 3,* 11, 50-54.

Living with low vision: A resource guide for people with sight loss. (1990). Lexington, MA: Resources for Rehabilitation.

Lloyd, J. H. (1984). Use of telescopic aids for vocational purposes. *Journal of Visual Impairment and Blindness, 78,* 5, 216-220.

Miller-Wood, D., Efron, M., & Wood, T. (1990). Use of closed-circuit television with a severely visually impaired young child. *Journal of Visual Impairment and Blindness, 84,* 10, 559-565.

Muranaka, Y., Furuta, N., Aoki, S., & Gohke, K. (1985). Use of the simplified color video magnifier by young children with severely impaired vision. *Journal of Visual Impairment and Blindness, 79,* 9, 319-395.

Potenski, D. (1983). Use of black light in training retarded, multiply handicapped, deaf-blind children. *Journal of Visual Impairment and Blindness, 77,* 7, 347-348.

Scholl, G. T. (Ed.). (1986). Low vision and visual efficiency. In *Foundations of education for blind and visually handicapped children and youth: Theory and practice.* New York: American Foundation for the Blind.

Sicurella, V. J. (1977). Color contrast as an aid for visually impaired persons. *Journal of Visual Impairment and Blindness, 71,* 6, 252-257.

Silberman, R. K. & Sowell, V. (1987). The visually impaired students with learning disabilities: Strategies for success in language arts. *Education of the Visually Handicapped, 18,* 4, 139-150.

Stratton, J. M. (1990). The principle of least-restrictive materials. *Journal of Visual Impairment and Blindness, 84,* 1, 3-5.

Watson, G. (1989). Competencies and a bibliography addressing students' use of low vision devices. *Journal of Visual Impairment and Blindness, 83,* 3, 160-163.

Wiener, W. & Vopata, A. (1980). Suggested curriculum for distance vision training with optical aids. *Journal of Visual Impairment and Blindness, 74,* 2, 49-56.

Medical Information Related to Visual Impairment

The Anatomy of the Eye

When reading a student's report, unfamiliar or forgotten terms may appear. The following description is a brief review of the parts of the eye and their role in the process of vision.

The **aqueous** is a clear, watery fluid that fills the anterior and posterior chambers of the eye (both posterior and anterior chambers are located in the front part of the eye, in front of the lens). It carries nutrients, removes waste products excreted from the lens, and helps to maintain the shape of the eye.

The **canal of schlemm** is a circular channel at the junction of the iris and the innermost layer of the cornea. The aqueous leaves the eye through this channel, and is absorbed by the aqueous veins.

The **choroid** is the middle layer of the eye between the sclera and the retina. It contains blood vessels that furnish nourishment to the other parts of the eye, especially the retina. The choroid is part of the uveal tract.

The **ciliary body** is a ring of tissue between the end of the choroid and the beginning of the iris. It is an extension of the choroid and part of the uveal tract. Part of the ciliary body produce the aqueous fluid, while another part controls the shape of the lens.

The **cones** are photoreceptive cells in the retina. They are concentrated in the macula area, and are responsible for both color perception and detail vision.

The **conjunctiva** is a delicate mucous membrane which lines the eyelids and covers all of the visible parts of the eye, except the cornea.

The **cornea** is the clear, transparent extension of the sclera. It is curved and is located in the front of the eye. It protects the inner contents of the eye and serves as a converging lens as the light passes through it. In coordination with the lens, it focuses light rays on the retina.

The **fovea centralis** is the center of the macula. It is a small depressed area and is composed entirely of cones. It is responsible for the sharpest central acuity and is the most light-sensitive area of the eye.

The **iris** is a forward extension of the ciliary body. It is a circular muscle in front of the lens. It controls the size of the pupil through which light enters the eye.

The **lens** is a colorless transparent oval structure suspended behind the iris. The lens changes its shape (between elongated and round) in order to focus light rays on the retina.

The **macula** is the area in the center of the retina that is primarily rod free. It is the area of clear central vision.

The **optic disc** (also called the blind spot) is the head of the optic nerve. It is formed by the meeting of the retinal tissue which becomes the optic nerve.

The **optic nerve** begins in the retina as the optic disk and carries messages from the rods and cones of the retina to the brain. These messages are interpreted in the brain and result in visual images.

The **pupil** is the opening in the center of the iris which appears as a black circle. Light enters the eye through the pupil.

The **retina** is the innermost layer of the eye. It contains light-sensitive nerve cells (photoreceptors) and fibers. It receives the image and sends it to the brain through the optic nerve.

The **rods** are photoreceptors in the retina. They are located primarily in the peripheral areas of the retina, and are responsible for seeing shape and motion. They are not receptive to color.

The **sclera** is the white part of the eye. It is a tough covering which forms a protective coating for all of the eyeball except for the cornea.

The **uveal tract** is composed of the choroid, the ciliary body, and the iris. It is the middle vascular layer of the eye protected externally by the cornea and the sclera which contributes to the blood supply of the retina.

The **vitreous** is a transparent colorless mass of soft gelatinous material which fills the globe of the eye between the lens and the retina. It maintains the shape of the eyeball. It must remain transparent in order for light to pass through it to the retina.

These parts of the eye can be grouped together into three layers :
The **outer protective layer -** sclera, cornea
The **middle vascular layer -** choroid, ciliary body, iris (This is often called the uveal tract.)
The **inner nerve layer -** retina, macula, fovea centralis, and by extension, the optic nerve)

The eye has three chambers:
The **anterior chamber** is between the cornea and the iris.
The **posterior chamber** is behind the iris and in front of the lens.
The **vitreous cavity** is the area behind the lens.

Light travels through the cornea, through the anterior chamber filled with aqueous, through the pupil and posterior chamber, through the lens, through the vitreous to the light-sensitive nerve cells (photoreceptors) in the retina.

Visual processing begins in the retina. Light energy produces chemical changes in the retina's light sensitive cells. These cells in turn, produce electrical activity which is communicated to the visual cortex of the brain by way of the optic nerve.

The visual cortex makes sense of the electrical impulses, and either files the information for future reference or sends a message to some motor area for action.

A visual impairment can result from interference with the passage of light through the eye, from interference with the focusing mechanism, from an inability of the retina to receive and change the energy from light to electrical form, from a difficulty in the transmission system from the retina to the brain, or in the brain's inability to receive and interpret the images transmitted.

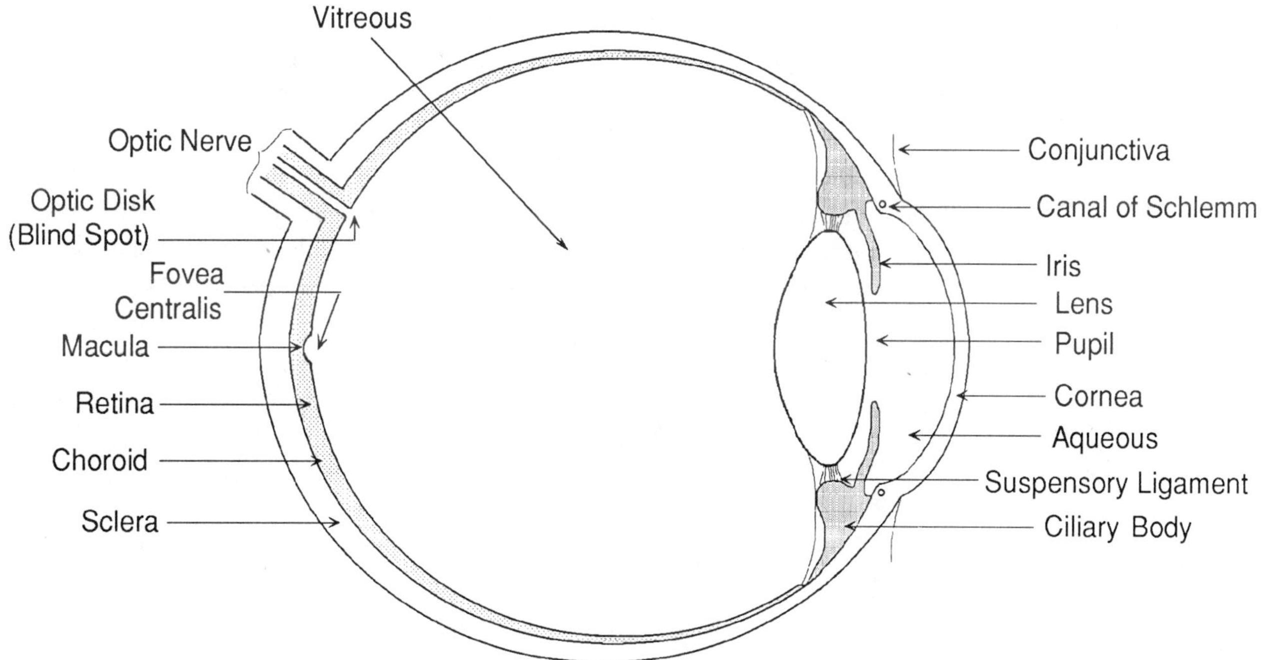

From Publication 169, National Society for the Prevention of Blindness, New York

It is important to understand the normal sequences of visual development. Only by understanding what is normal, can we identify what is abnormal. The Outline of Visual Abilities on pages 110 to 113 offers a progressive development of optical abilities, visual motor skills, and visual perceptual skills (visual discrimination, visual closure, visual sequencing, visual memory/visual imagery, figure-ground perception). When looking at this sequence of skills, it is clear that vision is made up of more than the optical system. The brain and the motor system must work with the eyes in order for vision to be most effective. The visual system will more nearly approximate the students' over-all developmental levels than their chronological age. However it is also important to remember that sometimes other cognitive and motor abilities "compensate" for the nonfunctioning areas and students function visually in ways that would not be predictable. Students may be able to perform some visual tasks that would not be expected of them if one simply looked at their physical condition.

While there are exceptions to the rule, a general guideline would be that visual developmental levels are closely related to overall developmental levels. Therefore when the students are young and their over-all development is within the approximate range of their chronological age, it is reasonable to plan visual activities that promote the development of the sequence of visual skills. When students are severely delayed, visually dependent task training and adaptations may be a more functional way to approach visual efficiency.

When students are young and have cortical visual impairments, they might be able to benefit from training in these developmental skills. They may be able to use the plasticity of the brain, to "reprogram" itself during their early years. Be sure to review the Guidelines for Programming for Students with Cortical Visual Impairments on pages 16 and 17.

When making decisions about what kind of programming to pursue, a general recommendation might be to try a developmental approach while students are young (up to six years of age), particularly if they are developing at a level that is close to their chronological age, or if students have recently sustained a head injury or other insult to the brain. However, when students are severely developmentally delayed, older than seven, or have shown little progress when working on visual skills in a developmental sequence, the instructor should seriously consider more functional visual programming. It is very important that an instructor not get "stuck" working on a very early developmental skill (such as tracking a light) when a student is ten years old and has shown little progress in this area. This student needs a more functional approach that focuses on specific visual needs in the activities that she is currently doing.

It is also important to point out that even when training within a developmental sequence is appropriate for the students involved, the activities should be meaningful and functional.

The following sequence of visual abilities has been adapted from "Development of Efficiency in Visual Functioning: Rationale for a Comprehensive Program" (Barraga & Collins, 1979a) and "Step-By-Step Charts: Sequence of Visual Development" (Ferrell, 1987), as well as other developmental sequences of skills. Whenever information was available, an estimated age has been added which suggests when children with vision that is functioning normally might develop these skills. However, it is important to keep in mind that these ages are estimations and some skills may be developed earlier than noted, and others may develop later among children who are still developing visual abilities within a normal pattern. The sequence of skill development may also differ among some children.

Optical Abilities

Simple responding
- Respond to a light source. (0-1 month)
- Respond to faces. (0-1 month)
- Respond to objects. (1-2 months)

Attending
- Briefly gaze at lights, objects and people that are nearby. (0-2 months)
- Visually attend to the actions of others. (1-3 months)

Shifting gaze and focus
- Shift gaze from one near object to another near object. (2-4 months)
- Visually examine and explore the environment. (2-4 months)
- Shift gaze and focus from a near object to a far object and from a far object to a near object. (3-5 months)

Tracking
- Track slowly moving lights, objects, and faces horizontally to midline and vertically. (1-3 months)
- Track horizontally across midline, and diagonally. (4-6 months)
- Track the movement of people within the immediate environment. (4-6 months)
- Visually follow the trajectory of a dropped object. (4-6 months)
- Visually follow an object as it goes behind him/her. (5-8 months)

Visual Motor

- Visually observe own personal movements. (4-8 months)

Facilitating gross motor movement
- Locate an object and move toward it. (4-8 months)
- Locate people and objects to be avoided when moving toward a goal and locate a path visually and move through it. (7-12 months)
- Imitate a variety of body movements. (7-12 months)
- Use vision to coordinate gross motor activities and make judgements about them. (10-18 months)

Pointing
- Visually locate objects pointed to by another person. (9-12 months)
- Point to objects within reach. (12-18 months)
- Point to objects in the environment. (12-18 months)

Facilitating fine motor tasks
- Use vision to reach for and grasp objects accurately. (5-7 months)
- Place an object in an open container or other designated location. (12-18 months)
- Fit objects together using visual cues. (12-24 months)
- Scribble within a designated space. (18-24 months)
- Match familiar objects using visual cues. (18 months -3 years)
- Imitate placement of objects after visual observation. (2-3 years)
- Use vision to coordinate fine motor activities and make judgements about them. (3 years)

Facilitating complex visual motor tasks
- Complete form boards, simple puzzles, or peg board designs. (2-3 years)
- Replicate a three-dimensional model through visual imitation. (2-3 years)
- Color a simple picture. (3-4 years)
- Connect dots to form a line or simple shape. (3-4 years)
- Copy simple marks or shapes. (3-4 years)
- Trace simple shapes and objects. (3-4 years)
- Cut between lines and on a broad line. (4-5 years)
- Cut out simple outlines and pictures. (4-5 years)

Visual Discrimination

Demonstrating an awareness of familiar objects and people
- Recognize familiar people visually. (1-3 months)
- Recognize familiar objects visually. (3-4 months)

Identifying shapes, drawings, and pictures
- Recognize self and others in a mirror or photograph. (18-24 months)
- Name simple outline pictures of familiar objects. (2-3 years)
- Select single elements in a picture. (2-3 years)
- Identify a variety of objects in pictures. (2-3 years)
- Match simple pictures or designs by inner detail. (3-4 years)
- Match similar pictures or objects when rotated. (3-5 years)
- Identify colors. (4-5 years)

Visual Closure

- Identify common objects regardless of minor structural changes. (2-3 years)
- Identify common objects which are partially hidden in the environment. (2-3 years)
- Identify objects partially hidden in pictures. (2-4 years)

Visual Sequencing

- Follow a given pattern. (3-4 years)
- Sequence several items by a given attribute (e. g., shape, size or color). (4 years)
- Arrange a set of pictures to tell a story. (4 years)

Visual Memory and Visual Imagery

Remembering a setting or location
- Recognize a change in a familiar room or setting. (18-24 months)
- Retrieve a toy from the place that it was last seen. (2-3 years)
- Identify missing objects. (3 years)
- Identify how objects or environments are similar and different. (3-4 years)

Describing details
- Describe familiar objects or environments. (3-4 years)
- Describe details in pictures and drawings. (4-5 years)

Drawing
- Draw a figure or a person. (4 years)
- Draw recognizable pictures of familiar objects or activities. (4-5 years)

Figure-Ground Perception

- Locate a specific object from a group of dissimilar objects. (1 year)
- Locate a specific object against a cluttered background. (1 year)
- Locate a specific object from a group of similar objects. (2 years)
- Select an object when only a part of it is visible. (2 years)
- Select an object when there is a similar background. (2 years)
- Locate a specific object in a cluttered environment or against a similar background. (3-4 years)
- Select a named object among several objects with similar configurations or from a group of similar objects when only a part of it is visible. (3-4 years)
- Select a named object or picture from a background containing moderate detail. (3-4 years)

GENETIC CONDITIONS

While the genetic factor in many eye diseases has been reasonably well established, the risk of occurrence can be predicted for some of these conditions, but others still cannot be predicted with any degree of accuracy.

Hereditary eye conditions are transmitted from parents to children in the following way. Genes which are contained within chromosomes, contain hereditary factors which determine body characteristics (as well as tendencies toward or manifestations of defects or diseases). Each person has forty-six chromosomes (twenty-three from each parent). Twenty-two of these chromosomes are called autosomes, and one is a sex chromosome, sometimes called X-linked. Each characteristic is represented in a pair of chromosomes (one element from each parent). Each pair can be a combination of two dominant traits, two recessive traits, or one dominant and one recessive trait. For example, in the autosomes, if *A* is a dominant trait and *a* is a recessive trait, the combinations could be *AA* (dominant), *aa* (recessive), or *Aa* (a combination in which the dominant trait prevails and the person *shows* the dominant trait and *carries* the recessive trait).

Therefore the term **autosomal dominant** means that a dominant characteristic has been transmitted through the autosomes, and **autosomal recessive** means that a recessive or "hidden" characteristic has been transmitted through the autosomes. **X-linked** means that a characteristic has been transmitted through the sex chromosome.

In **autosomal dominant inheritance**, if one parent exhibits a dominant characteristic, there is a 50% chance that the child will inherit it. If both parents exhibit the characteristic, the chance of inheriting it rises to 75%. Since there is no way of knowing whether the parent who shows the characteristic had a pair of genes that were both dominant, or had one dominant and one recessive gene, the probability is unclear unless an genetic study has been done on both parents.

In **autosomal recessive inheritance**, at least one parent can show the characteristic (i. e. , have both recessive genes for that characteristic), or both parents can carry the recessive gene. The child has a 50% chance of carrying the recessive gene if one parent shows it, and a 25% chance if neither parent shows it, but both parents carry it . Again there is no way to tell if a parent carries a recessive gene unless genetic studies have been done.

In **X-linked inheritance**, female parents who are carriers can pass on the characteristic or disease to their sons 50% of the time. Only males will be affected and fathers cannot pass on the characteristics to their sons.

Multifactorial genetic conditions are caused by the interaction of many genes with other genes or other environmental factors.

Also, entire chromosomes (the carriers of the genes) can be missing, as in Turner's syndrome, or extra chromosomes can be present, as in the trisomy disorders: Down's syndrome, Patau's syndrome, or Edward's syndrome.

Autosomal dominant - *forms of glaucoma, neurofibromatosis, retino-blastoma, colobomas, Marfan's syndrome, Sturge-Weber syndrome*

Examples of Hereditary Ocular Defects or Diseases

Autosomal recessive - *Crouzon's syndrome, keratoconus, myopia, Bassen-Kornzweig syndrome, Laurence-Moon-Biedl syndrome, Stargardt-Behr disease, Usher's syndrome, Leber's congenital amaurosis, galactosemia, Hurler's syndrome, Hermansky-Pudlac syndrome*

X-linked - *albinism, choroideremia, color blindness, Leber's disease, Loewe's syndrome, Norrie's disease*

Multifactorial - *diabetic retinopathy, glaucoma, strabismus, macular de-generation*

Chromosomal abnormalities - *Patau's syndrome, Edward's syndrome, Down's syndrome, Turner's syndrome, Cri-du-chat syndrome*

Some ocular defects may be so varied that they may be dominant, recessive, or X-linked (e. g., optic atrophy, retinitis pigmentosa), and some occur in families but their exact hereditary determination is unclear. (e. g., cataracts, glaucoma). Moreover, a number of eye defects occur as secondary symptoms of other diseases or syndromes (e. g., cataracts, glaucoma, retinitis pigmentosa,).

If a genetic factor is suspected, genetic counselling is recommended. See pages 48 and 49 for additional information.

SYNDROMES WHICH IMPACT EYE CONDITIONS

There are numerous syndromes or groups of symptoms that include eye disorders. The following chart lists many that students who are eligible for school programming might have. While the primary characteristics of the syndrome are listed, the primary emphasis is on the effect that the syndrome has on students' visual abilities.

Bassen-Kornzweig syndrome (abetalipoproteinemia)

An inherited disorder in which fat is not properly used causing degeneration of the light sensitive cells in the periphery of the retina, night blindness, tunnel vision, decreased acuity, and photophobia. It may lead to total blindness and damage to the central nervous system. It is a rare form of retinitis pigmentosa. Can be reversed in the early stages with large doses of vitamin A.

Batten-Vogt Mayou disease (neuronal ceroid-lipofuscinosis)

Pigmentary retinopathy, involving the macula most severely, causes loss of central vision, optic atrophy, and seizures. Occurs between ages five and ten.

CHARGE Association

Colobomas ranging from an isolated iris coloboma with no related visual impairment to clinical anophthalmos. Retinal coloboma is most common. It may also include heart disease, absence of the opening between the nasal cavity and the back of the throat, retarded growth and development and central nervous system abnormalities.

Coat's disease (Leber's miliary aneurysms)

A malformation of the retinal blood vessels, causing dilations and leakage in the peripheral retina leading to retinal detachment. It usually occurs in male children and young adults.

Cri-du-chat syndrome

A chromosomal defect that can cause retardation, microcephaly, hypotonia, strabismus, myopia, glaucoma, microphthalmus, coloboma, optic atrophy, and corneal opacity.

Crouzon's syndrome (craniofacial dysostosis)

A rare hereditary deformity (autosomal dominant) causing exophthalmos, enlargement of the nasal bones, abnormal increase in space between the eyes, optic atrophy, strabismus and nystagmus.

De Grouchy's syndrome

A chromosomal defect which causes ptosis, strabismus, myopia, glaucoma, microphthalmus, coloboma, optic atrophy, and corneal opacity as well as retardation, microcephaly, and midface hypoplasia.

De Morsier's syndrome (septo optic dysplasia)

A congenital brain malformation (absense of the septum pelucidum) characterized by shortness of stature, nystagmus, and optic nerve hypoplasia.

Down's syndrome (Trisomy 21)

A chromosomal abnormality causing high refractive errors, strabismus, nystagmus, esotropia, cataracts, keratoconus, moderate to severe developmental delays, possible cardiac abnormalities and distinct physical characteristics.

Duane's syndrome

A genetic (usually autosomal recessive) unilateral or bilateral eye muscle problem in the ability to move the eye(s) horizontally. The visual impairment is seldom severe.

Edward's syndrome (Trisomy 18)

A chromosomal abnormality (autosomal dominant) causing ptosis, corneal opacities, microphthalmus, glaucoma, uveal colobomas, hypopigmentation of the skin and hair, decreased growth, retardation, congenital heart disease, cleft lip and palate. Most children die within the first year.

Galactosemia

An autosomal recessive deficiency of the enzyme that processes galactose causing sugar cataracts, liver and spleen enlargement and developmental delays. Can be reversed if treated with a galactose-free diet.

Goldman-Favre syndrome

A rare disorder causing peripheral retinoschisis.

Hallerman-Streiff-François syndrome

A congenital condition that causes mandibular hypoplasia, feeding problems, and cataracts that mature rapidly in infancy.

Hermansky-Pudlac syndrome

An autosomal recessive form of albinism.

Hurler's syndrome (Gargoylism)

An inherited disorder (autosomal recessive) in which carbohydrates are not digested properly. Causes skeletal deformities, especially to the face, dwarfism, enlarged spleen and liver, and progressive physical and mental deterioration. The corneas show a diffuse haziness which progress to a white opacity. Other signs include slight ptosis, larger thickened eyelids, strabismus (esotropia), and glaucoma. Death usually occurs before ten years of age.

Laurence-Moon-Bardet-Beidel syndrome

An autosomal recessive disorder characterized by degeneration of the light sensitive cells in the periphery of the retina causing night blindness, tunnel vision, decreased acuity, and photophobia. Neurological progressive central field loss and photophobia may occur. Other conditions include obesity, hypogonadism, developmental delays, spastic paraplegia, and renal disorders.

Loewe's syndrome (oculocerebrorenal)

An X-linked recessive disorder causing severe eye involvement including cataracts, microphakia, and congenital glaucoma, as well as mental and growth retardation with hypotonia and usually early death.

Marchesani's syndrome

A rare hereditary disorder characterized by multiple skeletal and eye abnormalities including dislocated lens, myopia, glaucoma (which resists treatment) and poor prognosis for vision.

Marfan's syndrome

An autosomal dominant connective tissue disease which causes dislocated lens, strabismus, severe refractive errors, cataracts, secondary glaucoma, uveal colobomas, retinal detachments, and multiple pupils. It is characterized by increased length in the long bones of the arms, legs, fingers and toes, scanty subcutaneous fat, cardiovascular problems, and muscular underdevelopment.

Möbius' syndrome

A disorder which causes paralysis on both sides of the face causing lack of horizontal eye movements, other nervous system disorders, speech problems, and other defects of arms and legs.

Norrie's disease (atrophia bulborum hereditaria)

An X-linked, recessive disorder consisting of bilateral blindness from retinal detachment. Mental retardation and deafness can possibly develop later.

Patau's syndrome (Trisomy 13)

A congenital condition causing microphthalmos, colobomas, cataracts, retinal dysplasia, corneal opacities, optic nerve hypoplasia, as well as congenital heart disease, hernias, mental retardation, seizures, deafness, and microcephaly. Life expectancy is usually only a few months.

Peter's anomaly (Anterior chamber cleavage syndrome)

Central corneal opacity and adhesions on the iris and cornea which usually result in glaucoma.

Refsum's disease

An inborn error of metabolism causing retinal pigment epithelium degeneration, nystagmus, ptosis, small pupils, and possibly nerve deafness; a form of retinitis pigmentosa.

Reiter's syndrome

A triad of symptoms of unknown etiology comprising of urethritis (an infection of the urethra often causing bladder and kidney infections), conjunctivitis, and arthritis (the dominant feature). It is usually found in men and there is no satisfactory treatment.

Rubella syndrome

When the German measles virus is transmitted to the fetus by the mother during pregnancy. It can cause damage to the eyes, ears, heart, and brain. Eye damage can include congenital glaucoma, congenital cataracts, microphthalmus, decreased visual acuity, colobomas, nystagmus, strabismus, and constricted visual fields.

Scheie's syndrome

An autosomal recessive disorder which causes corneal clouding, and sometimes retinal pigmentary degeneration and optic atrophy.

Speilmeyer-Batten-Vogt disease

An autosomal recessive determined enzyme deficiency which results in pooling fats in the brain (lipid storage disease). Severe mental and physical deterioration occurs causing death within a few years. Optic atrophy and retinal pigmentary changes also occur.

Stargardt-Behr disease

An autosomal recessive disease causing pigmentary change in the macula resulting in a large scotoma in the central field of vision and nystagmus which usually occurs between the ages of six and twenty.

Stevens-Johnson syndrome (erythema multiforme major)

A disease of the mucous membranes and the skin causing bilateral conjunctivitis, ocular lesions, iritis, uveitis, corneal ulcers and photophobia. It may lead to corneal scarring and blindness. Pulmonary, renal, intestinal, and cardiac involvement may occur and may lead to death in severe forms.

Still's disease (Juvenile rheumatoid arthritis)

A form of rheumatoid arthritis that usually affects the larger joints of children under the age of sixteen and is more commonly found in girls. Accompanying eye complications include uveitis (iridiocyclitis), strabismus, cataracts, secondary glaucoma, and macular edema.

Sturge-Weber syndrome (encephalotrigeminal angiomatosis)

A congenital disease of the nerves of the skin characterized by port-wine noncancerous tumors on the face and eyes. It can cause infantile glaucoma, multicolored irises, seizures, contra-lateral hemiplegia, and intracranial calcification.

Tay-Sach's disease

A genetically determined (autosomal recessive) enzyme deficiency which results in pooling fats in the brain causing severe mental and physical deterioration. Vision begins deteriorating around six or seven months of age, and blindness usually occurs by eighteen months. Most children die between two and four years of age.

Turner's syndrome

A chromosomal abnormality marked by the absence of one X-chromosome which is found in females. It can cause dwarfism, ptosis, strabismus, blue sclera, eccentric pupils, cataracts, color deficiency, coloboma, as well as abnormal development of reproductive organs, spatial confusion, and learning disorders.

Usher's syndrome

> An autosomal recessive condition which causes hearing loss and degeneration of the peripheral vision.

Zellweger's syndrome (Cerebra hepatorenal syndrome)

> An autosomal recessive condition which causes "Leopard spot" peripheral retinal pigmentation, cataracts, congenital glaucoma, and optic nerve hypoplasia, as well as severe retardation. Life expectancy is usually less than a year.

The following is an attempt to consolidate into one chart information from a variety of sources. It includes information about the conditions which can cause visual impairment including the physical characteristics and medical treatment, the effect on the student's vision, environmental adaptations, low vision devices that might be helpful, and other educational considerations related to the condition. It is hoped that this chart will provide instructors with an accessible reference which can be used when reading medical reports, performing low vision assessments, and planning the student's educational program.

It is important to note that students who have a certain condition may not manifest all the characteristics that are described in the chart and their condition may not be severe enough to need the adaptations and educational considerations. The instructor will need to evaluate how the information in this chart should be applied to individual students.

SPECIFIC EYE CONDITIONS AND DISEASES WITH CORRESPONDING ADAPTATIONS

Eye Condition	Physical Characteristics(•) Medical Treatment(✛) Cause (▲)	Possible Resulting Effect on Vision	Adaptations	Educational Considerations
Albinism	• Total or partial lack of pigment causing abnormal optic nerve development, may or may not affect the skin color. Can be complete or partial albinism or ocular albinism. May be sensitive to exposure to the sun. ▲ Hereditary: may be autosomal recessive or X-linked.	Decreased visual acuity, photophobia, high refractive error, astigmatism, nystagmus, central scotomas, and strabismus.	Magnification, moving close to the object viewed, high contrast, tinted lenses, sunglasses and eyeshades or a cap with a brim, diffused lighting coming from behind the student, reduction of glare, enhanced print, corrective lenses, magnifiers/telescopes for distant vision.	Lighting conditions will need to be controlled to ensure optimal classroom performance. Teacher should not stand in front of the window or the light source when teaching or speaking to the student. High contrast line markers or templates may be helpful for reading, finding math problems or locating other important information. Print copies of overheads may need to be provided. Eye fatigue may occur, especially when doing close work. Difficulty with depth perception may occur.

Amblyopia ex anopsia (Lazy eye)

- Reduced visual functioning in one eye which causes the student to use only one eye instead of both.
- With young children, eye exercises, occlusion or patching of one eye and surgery may help.
- ▲ Caused by disease, strabismus, unequal refractive errors (anisometropia), or opacities of the lens or cornea.

- Monocularity, some field loss, poor or absent depth perception, may develop blindness in one eye.

- Good contrast and glare reduction.

- Close work may result in loss of place, eye fatigue, blurring of print, poor concentration. Frequent rest periods may be needed when doing close work. Classroom seating should favor the student's functional eye. The student may have difficulty with inaccurate reach with steps and drop-offs and other physical activities, and may need more time to adjust to new situations. Familiarization with the environment can ease the awkwardness and help to anticipate distances and heights.

Aniridia

- Total or partial absence of the iris. Often patients with aniridia have **Wilm's Tumor.**
- ▲ Hereditary: usually is autosomal dominant, but could be autosomal recessive as well.

- Decreased visual acuity, photophobia, and field loss which corresponds to the areas where the iris is absent. Cataracts and glaucoma are frequently present. Vision may fluctuate depending on lighting conditions and glare.

- Cosmetic contact lenses which create an artificial pupil, tinted lenses, sunglasses and eyeshades, dim lighting, rheostats and lighting controls, magnification.

- Lighting conditions will need to be controlled to ensure optimal classroom performance. Teacher should not stand in front of the window or the light source when teaching or speaking to the student. Print copies of overhead transparencies can be helpful. Give extra time to adapt to change in lighting. Be sensitive to eye fatigue.

Eye Condition	Physical Characteristics(•) Medical Treatment(✛) Cause (▲)	Possible Resulting Effect on Vision	Adaptations	Educational Considerations
Anophthalmos, Anophthalmia	• Absence of one or both eyeballs. ▲ Hereditary, associated with chromosomal variation.	Total blindness, if both eyes are affected.	Prosthetic eyes	If both eyes are effected, tactual and auditory modes will be used.
Aphakia	• Absence of the lens, usually caused when the lens is surgically removed due to cataracts.	Inability to accommodate, may have depth perception problems.	Contact lenses, good contrast and lighting, magnification, enlargement or bringing items closer to the eyes.	Lights with rheostats and adjustable arms are helpful for close work. Sunvisors can be worn indoors. If contact lenses or glasses are prescribed, they should be worn.
Astigmatism	• A defect in the curvature of the cornea; light rays cannot focus on a single point on the retina. ▲ May be hereditary.	Blurred vision, commonly occurs with albinism and keratoconus, tendency to frown to create a "pinhole effect".	Corrective lenses, good contrast and lighting.	May tire easily and complain of headaches when reading and doing close work.
Buphthalmos (Infantile glaucoma)	• A form of glaucoma that has its outset at birth or within the first three years. ✛ Surgery ▲ Hereditary: usually autosomal recessive.	Photophobia, increased ocular pressure, tearing, damage to the optic disc, increased corneal diameter, corneal opacity, increased depth of the anterior chamber, as well as general enlargement of the anterior chamber of the eye. Blindness occurs if left untreated.	If any vision remains, good contrast and lighting may be helpful.	If blindness occurs, tactual and auditory modes will need to be developed.

6.

Cataracts

- Opacity or cloudiness of the lens which restricts the passage of light, usually bilateral. Immature or incipient cataracts are only slightly opaque; while mature cataracts are so opaque that the fundus cannot be seen and the pupil may be white.

✛ Surgical removal is usually recommended when the cataract becomes mature. Intraocular lens (IOL) implants or corneal contact lenses may be used after surgery.

▲ Caused by injury or trauma, drugs, malnutrition or rubella during pregnancy, aging, some eye diseases (e. g., uveitis, glaucoma, retinitis pigmentosa, retinal detachment) and heredity. May be autosomal dominant or X-linked.

➠ Reduced acuity, blurred vision, poor color vision, photophobia, and sometimes nystagmus. Visual ability fluctuates according to light. Squint or strabismus may be early manifestations of congenital cataracts. Amblyopia may result if not corrected. After surgery the eye(s) cannot accommodate without lens prescriptions.

👁 Magnification, enlargement or bringing the materials closer to the eyes. Eccentric viewing may be helpful. Lighting should come from behind the student and glare should be avoided. If cataracts are centrally located, near vision will be affected and bright light may be a major problem. Low level of illumination may be preferred. If cataracts are in the peripheral area, bight light may be needed to close the pupil and allow the iris to cover most of the cataract area. If the lens has been removed, see aphakia.

✎ Teacher should not stand in front of the window or the light source when teaching or speaking to the student. Lights with rheostats and adjustable arms are helpful for close work. If contact lenses or glasses are prescribed, they should be worn. Time may be needed for adjustment to different lighting situations. Rest periods may be needed when doing close work and variation of near and distant tasks can prevent tiring

Eye Condition	Physical Characteristics(•) Medical Treatment(✝) Cause (▲)	Possible Resulting Effect on Vision	Adaptations	Educational Considerations
Chorioretinitis	• Posterior uveitis or an inflammation of the choroid that spreads to the retina. ▲ Can be caused by tuberculosis, histoplasmosis, or toxoplasmosis.	Can cause blurred vision, photophobia, distorted images, central scotomas.	Eccentric viewing, magnification to enlarge the image beyond the scotoma, enlargement of materials or bringing materials closer to the eye, diffused less intense light may permit the eyes to enlarge the pupil so more area can be viewed, telescopes for distance vision, tinted glasses, sunglasses and eyeshades, closed-circuit television with reversed polarity, adjustable lighting without glare.	High contrast line markers or templates may be helpful for reading, finding math problems or locating other important information.
Choroideremia	• Degeneration of pigment and retinal atrophy. ▲ Hereditary: X-linked.	In males, night blindness, constricted visual field, progressive blindness. In females, nonprogressive, normal vision, often an atypical retinopathy.	Diffused lighting with no glare, absorptive lenses, infra-red viewing devices, prism glasses to increase visual field, closed circuit television for maximum contrast, reversed polarity.	Physical activities and mobility may be restricted by low light situations such as bad weather and nighttime. Teach organized search patterns using a "grid" pattern to aid the student in locating objects or visual targets. Students may need to be seated farther away to increase their visual field.

Coloboma

● A birth defect which causes a notch or cleft in the pupil, iris, ciliary body, lens, retina, choroid or optic nerve which occurs during fetal development. A "keyhole pupil" often occurs. ▲ Hereditary: autosomal dominant.	➠ Decreased acuity, photophobia, nystagmus, strabismus; field loss occurs if it extends to the retina. Cataracts, refractive errors and problems with depth perception may occur. Glaucoma can develop in later life.	⊖ Magnification, average or bright light with no glare, cosmetic contact lenses which create an artificial pupil, telescopes for distance viewing, sunglasses and eyeshades if the coloboma is in the iris.	✎ High contrast line markers or templates may be helpful for reading, finding math problems or locating other important information.

Color Deficiency or Color Blindness

● Cone malformation, macular deficiency, partial or total absence of cones. ▲ Hereditary: X-linked or caused by retinal disease or poisoning.	➠ Difficulty or the inability to see colors and detail, photophobia, nystagmus, macular deficiencies, central field scotomas, normal peripheral fields.	⊖ High contrast, tinted lenses, sunglasses or eyeshades, diffused illumination without glare.	✎ Avoid activities dependent on color or discrimination. Alternative techniques for interpreting color will need to be taught (e. g., the position of the red and green lights in a traffic signal, using color identification tags on clothing).

Cone Monochromacy (See Color Deficiency)

Eye Condition	Physical Characteristics(•) Medical Treatment(✛) Cause (▲)	Possible Resulting Effect on Vision	Adaptations	Educational Considerations
Conjunctivitis	• An inflammation of the conjunctiva, most common eye disease of the Western Hemisphere, causing red, painful, irritated eyes, tearing and discharge. ✛ Depending on the cause, medication is usually prescribed. ▲ Caused by bacteria, chlamydia, virus, fungus, parasites, allergies, and chemical irritants. Associated with thyroid disease and gout.	➡ Photophobia, may cause corneal ulcers and scarring, ptosis, refractive errors, and can lead to blindness in some cases.	👁 Lighting should come from behind the student and glare should be avoided.	✎ Rest periods may be needed when doing close work. Time may be needed to adjust to different lighting situations.

Corneal Opacities (See Corneal Ulcers)

Corneal Ulcers	• An open sore or scarring on the cornea. ✛ Medication and sometimes scraping or removing the ulcer. If scarring is extensive, a corneal transplant may be necessary. ▲ Caused by bacteria, viruses, fungi, vitamin deficiency, a hypersensitive reaction, or lack of tears.	➡ Can appear on any part of the cornea with resulting impairment, blurred vision, reduced central acuity, and can lead to blindness.	👁 Eccentric viewing, good lighting and contrast, magnification.	✎ Lights with rheostats and adjustable arms are helpful for close work.

Cortical Visual Impairment

- Damage to the visual cortex or the posterior visual pathways. Pervasive neurological disorders such as cerebral palsy, epilepsy, hydrocephalus, learning disabilities, or deafness may be present. Occasionally optic nerve atrophy, optic nerve hypoplasia, retinal abnormalities and other ocular lesions occur. Spatial confusion is common.

- Caused by anoxia at birth, a head injury, infections to the central nervous system (such as encephalitis and meningitis), shunt failure, or a genetic malformation.

- Fluctuation in visual functioning, eye structure may be healthy and intact, sometimes absence of nystagmus, inattention to visual stimuli, preference of touch over vision as the primary exploratory sense, difficulty seeing objects or pictures which are placed close together, difficulty discriminating figure-ground, may have more peripheral than central vision or vice versa. Color perception is generally intact. Visual improvement sometimes occurs over a period of time after the initial insult to the brain. Light gazing frequently occurs. Students may bring objects close to their eyes to block out the extraneous visual clutter in order to concentrate more easily on the object.

- High illumination, bright contrast in materials, using consistent visual cues throughout different settings such as school, home and the community. A combination of reading media may be necessary. See pages 48 and 49 for more discussion on considerations for programming.

- Most students who have a cortical visual impairment are also multiply impaired. It is necessary to determine which sensory system gives most accurate information to the student and then pair visual skills with that system. Visual input must be controlled to prevent "visual overloading". Visual images should be simple and presented in isolation. Repetition and routines are very helpful. Tell students what they are seeing and encourage them to feel it and explore it while learning about it. Color coding simple pictures or shapes gives an additional cue for recognition. Restrict the number of people who are directly involved in intervention. When preparing reading materials, use a contrasting paper, template or marker to block out some of the visual information, or space objects farther apart on a page Demonstrate how to use a finger to move from one object to the next on a page. Simplify illustrations. Fluctuations in visual performance may be reduced by eliminating tiredness, extraneous noise and other distractors. It may be necessary to turn off a light or use diffused lighting to get students to foucs on a task.

132

Eye Condition	Physical Characteristics(•) Medical Treatment(✛) Cause (▲)	Possible Resulting Effect on Vision	Adaptations	Educational Considerations
Diabetic Retinopathy	• Both juvenile onset and maturity onset diabetes can cause changes in the blood vessels of the retina causing hemorrhaging in the retina and vitreous, sensory loss in the feet and hands, and possible retinal detachment and blindness. ✛ Caused by diabetes mellitis. Dietary controls and insulin treatments may be needed to control the diabetes. ▲ Can be hereditary: multifactorial.	➡ Sensitivity to glare, double vision, lack of accommodation, fluctuating acuity, diminished color vision, defective visual fields, floating obstructions in the vitreous, retinal detachment. If hemorrhages recur, vision may fluctuate.	👓 Good lighting and contrast, magnification, closed circuit television.	✎ Stress and pressure to perform can negatively affect stabilization of blood glucose. Tactual sensation is often poor and reflexes can be slow. Diet can influence attentiveness. Students with advanced sensory loss in their hands and feet may not be able to read braille and may not sense drop offs.
Diplopia	• A defect in the muscles restricting the eyes' ability to work together causing "double vision". The image from one eye is imposed on the image from the other eye. If left untreated it can develop into amblyopia.	➡ Visual confusion or "double vision", dizziness, suppression occurs which results in monocular vision or amblyopia.	👓 Good contrast and glare reduction, more time to adjust to new situations. Corrective lenses may be helpful.	✎ Close work may result in loss of place, eye fatigue, blurring of print, poor concentration and headaches. Frequent rest periods may be needed when doing close work. Familiarization with the environment can ease the awkwardness and help to anticipate distances and heights.

Dislocated Lens

- The lens is not in its natural position.
- ✛ Often left untreated when there are no complications.
- ▲ Hereditary or caused by accident or trauma; sometimes associated with coloboma, Marfan's syndrome, or Marchesani's syndrome.

➡ Blurred vision, diplopia, cataracts.

👓 Good contrast and lighting.

✎ Close work may result in loss of place, eye fatigue, blurring of print, poor concentration. Frequent rest periods may be needed when doing close work.

Enucleation

- The anterior chamber or the entire globe of the eye is surgically removed from the orbit.
- ✛ Prosthetic eyes or scleral shells are usually recommended.
- ▲ Caused by accident or trauma, malignancy, or severe pain or disfigurement in a blind eye.

➡ If one eye is removed, there is no depth perception. If the remaining eye is impaired, the condition is more serious.

👓 Prosthetic eyes. If one eye remains, good contrast and reduction of glare may help. More time may be needed to adjust to new situations.

✎ Lack of depth perception may result in inaccurate reach, and difficulty with steps and drop-offs. Familiarization with the environment can ease awkwardness and help to anticipate distances and heights. Classroom seating should favor the student's functional eye.

Eye Condition	Physical Characteristics(•) Medical Treatment(✛) Cause (▲)	Possible Resulting Effect on Vision	Adaptations	Educational Considerations
Glaucoma	• An eye disease which causes increased pressure in the eye because of blockage in the normal flow of the fluid in the aqueous humor. ✛ Eye drops are prescribed and must be used regularly to reduce pressure. Surgery may be needed. ▲ Caused by changes in the lens or uveal tract, trauma, reaction to certain medications, surgical procedures or heredity. If inherited: autosomal recessive, autosomal dominant, or multifactorial.	May cause fluctuating visual functioning, peripheral field loss, poor night vision, photophobia, difficulty reading or seeing large objects at close range, decreased sensitivity to contrast, pain or headaches, eye redness, hazy cornea, wide open pupil. Can lead to degeneration of the optic disc and blindness if untreated.	Sunglasses and eyeshades, lamps with rheostats or adjustable lighting to provide good quality lighting with no glare, good contrast, magnifiers, closed-circuit television, absorptive lenses.	Fluctuations in visual performance can be frustrating to the student. Expectations may need to be adjusted accordingly. Stress and fatigue have a negative effect on visual performance. Teachers should be alert to symptoms of pain and increased pressure. If medication is prescribed, it should be taken regularly. Travel in unfamiliar places may be difficult.
Histoplasmosis, Presumed Ocular Histoplasmosis Syndrome (POHS)	• Fungus infection causing retinal damage. ✛ Steroids are used to treat the initial infection.	Macula damage or central scotomas cause patchy fields, central vision loss and deficient color vision while peripheral damage causes loss of night vision. When the retinal damage is in the central area, see the adaptations and educational considerations in macular disease. When the damage is in the periphery, see the adaptations and educational considerations in retinitis pigmentosa.	Microscopes, telescopes, good contrast and lighting.	High contrast line markers or templates may be helpful for reading, finding math problems or locating other important information.

Hyperopia (Farsightedness)

- A refractive error in which the focal point for light rays is behind the retina; shortness of the eyeball. If not corrected, close work may cause nausea, headache, dizziness and eye rubbing.

➡ Difficulty seeing at close distances.

👓 Corrective lenses, magnifiers.

✎ Students may tire easily when reading and doing close work. Variation in near and far tasks can prevent tiring. Students may prefer physical education activities and activities that require distance vision.

Hypoplasia (See Optic Atrophy)

Keratitis (See Corneal Ulcer)

Keratoconus

- The cornea becomes cone shaped. Can be found with retinitis pigmentosa, Down's syndrome, Marfan's syndrome, and aniridia. Seems to be congenital and bilateral. Usually has onset in young adulthood.

+ Corneal transplants are often necessary.

▲ Seems to be inherited (autosomal recessive) but most cases do not show a definite genetic pattern.

➡ Decreased distance vision, astigmatism, sensitivity to glare, distortion of entire visual field, possible corneal rupture and can lead to blindness.

👓 Contact lenses are used to retard the bulging of the cornea in the early stages. Good contrast and lighting; avoid glare.

✎ Avoid activities that could cause corneal damage such as contact sports and swimming in heavily chlorinated water.

Eye Condition	Physical Characteristics(•) Medical Treatment(✛) Cause (▲)	Possible Resulting Effect on Vision	Adaptations	Educational Considerations
Leber's Congenital Amaurosis	• A form of retinitis pigmentosa causing degeneration of the macula occurring at or shortly after birth, progressive central field loss; abnormal corneas and cataracts may be present. ▲ Hereditary: autosomal recessive.	Central and peripheral vision can be affected; loss of color vision and detail, nystagmus is present. Excessive rubbing of eyes is characteristic.	Eccentric viewing using peripheral vision, magnification to enlarge the image beyond the scotoma, enlargement of materials or bringing materials closer to the eye, diffused less intense light may permit the eyes to enlarge the pupil so more area can be viewed, telescopes for distance vision, tinted glasses, sunglasses and eyeshades, closed-circuit television with reversed polarity, adjustable lighting without glare.	High contrast line markers or templates may be helpful for reading, finding math problems or locating other important information. Teachers should not stand in front of a window or light source when teaching or speaking to the student. Lights with rheostats and adjustable arms are helpful for close work. Fatigue can become a problem.
Leber's Optic Atrophy	• A rare disease characterized by rapidly progressive optic atrophy, which occurs in young men and rarely in women and may include other types of central nervous system involvement. ▲ Hereditary: X linked recessive.	Reduced central activity, fluctuating visual performance, blurred vision, color vision may be impaired; visual perception may be impaired.	High illumination, enlarged print, magnification, high contrast.	Avoid visual clutter; images should be simple and presented in isolation. When teaching avoid standing in front of a busy background and wearing busy patterns. Modify expectations to accommodate fluctuating visual performance.

17. **Macular Disease, Macular Degeneration (Age Related Macular Degeneration), Congenital Macular Disease**

- Progressive or degenerating damage to the central part of the retinal cones. Can be "juvenile" (occurring before the age of seven) or "senile".

▲ Hereditary: multifactorial.

➡ Affects central vision, photophobia, poor color vision, normal peripheral vision.

👓 Eccentric viewing using peripheral vision, magnification to enlarge the image beyond the scotoma, enlargement of materials or bringing materials closer to the eye, diffused less intense light may permit the eyes to enlarge the pupil so more area can be viewed, telescopes for distance vision, tinted glasses, sunglasses and eyeshades, closed-circuit television with reversed polarity, adjustable lighting without glare.

✎ High contrast line markers or templates may be helpful for reading, finding math problems or locating other important information. Teachers should not stand in front of a window or light source when teaching or speaking to the student. Lights with rheostats and adjustable arms are helpful for close work. Fatigue can become a problem. Students may need to be seated near the chalkboard.

18. **Microphthalmos, Microphthalmia**

- A congenital birth defect that causes one or both eyes to be abnormally small. May occur with other congenital abnormalities such as club foot, additional fingers or toes, webbed fingers or toes, polycystic kidneys, and cystic liver.

▲ Hereditary: most frequently recessive, sometimes dominant.

➡ Decreased visual acuity, photophobia, may have fluctuating visual abilities. May result in cataracts, glaucoma, aniridia, and coloboma.

👓 Average or bright light with no glare, good contrast, may need magnification.

✎ Fluctuations in visual performance can be frustrating to the student and expectations may need to be adjusted accordingly. Be alert for stress and fatigue.

Eye Condition	Physical Characteristics(●) Medical Treatment(✛) Cause (▲)	Possible Resulting Effect on Vision	Adaptations	Educational Considerations
Myopia (simple), Degenerative Myopia, (Nearsightedness)				
	● A refractive error where the image of a distant object is formed in front of the retina and cannot be seen distinctly; elongation of the eyeball. ✛ Surgery is experimental, but may be helpful in some cases. Screen for glaucoma. ▲ Hereditary: autosomal recessive.	⇒ Inability to see at distances. Near vision is rarely affected. Squinting and frowning may be indications of difficulty seeing things at a distance. **Degenerative myopia** can cause severe nearsightedness, is progressive and often visual acuity cannot be corrected to normal with lenses. Diagnosis is based on changes observed in the retina and the choroid. Detached retina, choroidal hemorrhages, reduced central vision, opacities of the vitreous, macular swelling, and cataracts can occur.	↢ Corrective lenses, high illumination with minimal glare, contact lenses.	✎ With degenerative myopia, students may need to move closer to see the blackboard and classroom demonstrations. Students who have progressive myopia should observe precautions for retinal detachment. Students may not be interested in activities that require distance vision, especially physical education activities.
Nystagmus	● Involuntary eye movements which can be horizontal, vertical, circular or mixed. Can be elicited when someone watches certain kind of moving objects. ✛ Muscle surgery may be helpful. ▲ Causes are often unknown but can be hereditary (autosomal recessive) or caused by neurological or inner ear disturbances.	⇒ Inability to maintain steady fixation, reduced visual acuity, fatigue, vertigo.	↢ Shifting gaze or head tilting may help to find the "null point" which slows the nystagmus.	✎ Stress and spinning or other rhythmic movements increase nystagmus, and should be avoided when visual functioning needs to be maximized. Close work causes fatigue and visual tasks should be varied to provide rest for the eyes. Line markers, rulers, typoscopes and other templates may be helpful to keep the place on the page. Good lighting and contrast are helpful.

21. **Optic Atrophy, Optic Nerve Atrophy**

- Dysfunction of the optic nerve resulting in the inability to conduct electrical impulses to the brain causing loss of vision. The optic disc becomes pale and there is a loss of pupillary reaction.

▲ Caused by disease, pressure on the optic nerve, trauma, glaucoma, toxicity or heredity; if inherited: dominant.

➡ Fluctuating visual performance, blurred vision, color vision may be impaired, visual perception may be impaired.

⚭ High illumination, enlarged print, magnification, high contrast; braille and tactual materials may be needed.

✎ Avoid visual clutter, images should be simple and presented in isolation. When teaching avoid standing in front of a busy background and wearing busy patterns. Modify expectations to accommodate fluctuating visual performance. Vision stimulation programming is essential for young children to help them learn how to interpret what they see.

22. **Optic Nerve Hypoplasia**

- A congenital non-progressive anomaly in which the optic nerve head appears small and grey or pale and is often surrounded by a mottled yellow halo bordered by a dark ring of pigment, called the "double ring sign". There is often indication of abnormalities of the midline structures of the visual system, such as the corpus callosum, causing midline deficiencies. There is often a dramatic asymmetry between the two optic heads. Central nervous system and endocrine anomalies, cerebral palsy and mental retardation also can occur.

▲ An insult to the prenatal central nervous system. Commonly found with fetal alcohol syndrome, frequently found in first born children of very young mothers. May be genetic and can be caused by trauma.

➡ Decreased visual acuity which may vary from light perception to normal acuity, variable field defects, nystagmus.

⚭ High illumination, enlarged print, magnification, high contrast; braille and tactual materials may be needed.

✎ Avoid visual clutter, images should be simple and presented in isolation. When teaching avoid standing in front of a busy background and wearing busy patterns. Modify expectations to accommodate fluctuating visual performance. Vision stimulation programming is essential for young children to help them learn how to interpret what they see.

Eye Condition	Physical Characteristics(•) Medical Treatment(✛) Cause (▲)	Possible Resulting Effect on Vision	Adaptations	Educational Considerations
Papilledemia	• A swelling of the optic disc caused by pressure in the skull; optic atrophy may occur. ▲ Caused by cerebral tumors, reaction to drugs, abscesses, subdural hematoma, or hydrocephalus.	➡ The blind spot is enlarged, but visual fields and visual acuity are otherwise normal. If optic atrophy occurs, slight to total loss of vision can result.	👓 If optic atrophy occurs, high illumination, enlarged print, magnification, high contrast.	✎ If optic atrophy occurs, avoid visual clutter; images should be simple and presented in isolation. When teaching, avoid standing in front of a busy background and wearing busy patterns. Modify expectations to accommodate fluctuating visual performance.
Presbyopia	• Gradual hardening of the lens which increases with age. ✛ Usually requires prescription lenses by the time people are in their mid-forties.	➡ Reduced ability to accommodate.	👓 Good lighting and contrast.	
Phthisis bulbi	• Abnormally low pressure of the eye which can cause shrinkage of the eye.	➡ May lead to total malfunction of the eye.	👓 Average or bright light with no glare, good contrast; may need magnification.	✎ High contrast line markers or templates may be helpful for reading, finding math problems or locating other important information. If blindness occurs, tactual and auditory modes will need to be developed.

Ptosis

- Drooping of the eyelid, may be unilateral or bilateral, constant or intermittent.
+ Medication may be called for with myasthenia gravis, surgery may be needed if the condition is severe.
▲ Caused by heredity, damages to the muscle or nerves, swelling or tumors.

➡ Reduced visual field may cause amblyopia.

👓 Frames can be worn that have a wire crutch that elevates the lid.

✎ Position and placement for activities may affect visual efficiency.

Retinal dysplasia

- Abnormal growth or development of the retina.

➡ Field loss, blurred vision, scotomas or blind spots, possibly loss of central vision.

👓 Magnification for close work, telescopes for distance viewing, eccentric viewing, high illumination, eliminate glare.

✎ If field loss occurs, physical activities and mobility may be restricted by low light situations such as bad weather or nighttime. Teach organized search patterns using a "grid" pattern to aid the student in locating objects or visual targets. Students may need to be seated farther away to increase their visual field. If loss of central vision occurs, teachers should not stand in front of a window or light source when teaching or speaking to the student. Lights with rheostats and flexible arms may be helpful for close work.

Eye Condition	Physical Characteristics(•) Medical Treatment(✛) Cause(▲)	Possible Resulting Effect on Vision	Adaptations	Educational Considerations
Retinal Detachment	• Parts of the retina pull away from the supporting structure of the eye and atrophy. ✛ The retina may be reattached if little time has transpired. ▲ Caused by diabetes, a blow to the head, trauma or degenerative myopia.	➡ Field loss, blurred vision, scotomas or blind spots, possibly loss of central vision; myopia and strabismus often occur when there is remaining vision. When the retinal detachment is in the central area, see the adaptations and educational considerations in macular disease. When the detachment is in the periphery, see the adaptations and educational considerations in retinitis pigmentosa.	👓 Magnification for close work, telescopes for distance viewing, eccentric viewing, high illumination. Eliminate glare.	✎ Avoid contact sports and any physical activity that may result in a sudden jar of the head to prevent further detachment.
Retinitis pigmentosa	• A progressive disorder that causes degeneration primarily of the light sensitive cells in the periphery of the retina. There are numerous diseases grouped together which damage the retina in this way but manifest additional different characteristics. These include: Usher's syndrome, Leber's congenital amaurosis, Laurence-Moon-Biedl syndrome, and Bassen-Kornzweig syndrome. ▲ Usually hereditary: autosomal dominant, autosomal recessive or X-linked.	➡ Loss of peripheral vision, night blindness, tunnel vision, decreased acuity and depth perception, spotty vision because of retinal scarring, and photophobia. Cataracts can develop. May be accompanied by myopia, vitreous opacities, cataracts, or keratoconus. Total blindness occurs in some cases.	👓 High illumination with no glare, absorptive lenses, infra-red viewing devices, prism glasses to increase visual field, closed circuit television for maximum contrast.	✎ Physical activities and mobility may be restricted by low light situations such as bad weather and nighttime. Teach organized search patterns using a "grid" pattern to aid the student in locating objects or visual targets. Students may need to be seated farther away to increase their visual field. Precautions should be taken to prevent retinal detachment.

25. **Retinoblastoma**

- A malignancy of the retina in early childhood which usually requires enucleation and can occur in one or both eyes.

+ Surgery, radiotherapy, chemotherapy, cryotherapy or photocoagulation may be helpful. Bilateral retinoblastoma has increased risk of developing other tumors. Regular physical examinations are encouraged.

▲ Hereditary: autosomal dominant.

➡ If one eye is removed, there is no depth perception. If the remaining eye is impaired, the condition is more serious. The first sign of the disease may be strabismus (esotropia or exotropia).

👓 Prosthetic eyes

✎ The absence of depth perception may result in inaccurate reach, and difficulty with steps and drop-offs. Students may have good spatial awareness due to early vision. Many have cognitive and academic abilities at the high and low extremes.

26. **Retinopathy of Prematurity (Retrolental fibroplasia)**

- A curtailment of retinal blood vessel development in premature infants which can lead to bleeding, scarring, and retinal detachment. Can range from minimal damage to complete blindness.

+ Treatments include Vitamin E therapy, photocoagulation procedures, cryotherapy, scleral buckling procedures, and vitrectomy, but none is totally successful. Some cases resolve themselves without intervention.

▲ Primary contributors are low birthweight, early gestational age, and duration and administration of oxygen.

➡ Decreased visual acuity, severe myopia, possible retinal detachment, spotty vision strabismus, retinal scarring, field loss, possible glaucoma.

👓 High illumination, magnification for close work, telescopes for distance viewing, closed-circuit television.

✎ Students may have brain damage resulting in behavior problems and/or developmental delays. Precautions should be taken to prevent retinal detachment. Early intervention and sensory stimulation are important.

Eye Condition	Physical Characteristics(•) Medical Treatment(✛) Cause (▲)	Possible Resulting Effect on Vision	Adaptations	Educational Considerations
Rod Monochromacy (Achromatopsia)	• Cones are absent or abnormal resulting in the absence of color vision. ▲ Hereditary: autosomal recessive or X-linked.	Poor visual acuity but near vision is usually better than distance vision. Nystagmus and photophobia improve with age. Colors are seen as shades of gray.	Tinted lenses, reduced lighting.	Student will not be able to perceive colors but may learn to make color judgements based on brightness. Alternative techniques for interpreting color will need to be taught (e.g., the position of the red and green lights in a traffic signal, using color identification tags on clothing).
Sclerosis	• A disease of the choroid leading to the slow loss of central vision in middle life. ▲ Hereditary: autosomal dominant or recessive.	Affects central vision, photophobia, poor color vision, normal peripheral vision.	Eccentric viewing, magnification to enlarge the image beyond the scotoma, enlargement of materials or bringing materials closer to the eye, diffused less intense light may permit the eyes to enlarge the pupil so more area can be viewed, telescopes for distance vision, tinted glasses, sunglasses and eyeshades, closed-circuit television with reversed polarity, adjustable lighting without glare.	High contrast line markers or templates may be helpful for reading, finding math problems or locating other important information.

Scotoma

- A portion of the visual field that is blind or partially blind.

➡ Affects central vision, photophobia, poor color vision, normal peripheral vision.

👓 Eccentric viewing, magnification to enlarge the image beyond the scotoma, enlargement of materials or bringing materials closer to the eye, diffused less intense light may permit the eyes to enlarge the pupil so more area can be viewed, telescopes for distance vision, tinted glasses, sunglasses and eyeshades, closed-circuit television with reversed polarity, adjustable lighting without glare.

✎ High contrast line markers or templates may be helpful for reading, finding math problems or locating other important information.

Eye Condition	Physical Characteristics(•) Medical Treatment(✛) Cause (▲)	Possible Resulting Effect on Vision	Adaptations	Educational Considerations
28. **Strabismus**	• The inability of both eyes to look directly at an object at the same time, a muscle imbalance, often secondary to other visual impairments. ✛ With young children, eye exercises, occlusion or patching of the good eye or surgery may help. ▲ Hereditary: multifactorial.	➠ Affects binocular vision, depth perception and eye-hand coordination. There are different types of strabismus: **esophoria** -a tendency for one or both eyes to turn inward, **esotropia** or "crossed eyes" - an inward deviation of one eye in relation to the other, **exophoria** - a tendency for one or both eyes to turn outward, **exotropia** or "walled eyes" - an outward deviation of one eye in relation to the other, **hypertropia** - a tendency for one or both eyes to turn upward, **hyperopheria** - a deviation of one eye upward, **hypophoria** - a tendency for one or both eyes to turn downward, and **hypotropia** - a tendency for one eye to turn downward lower than the other. May cause eye-strain and difficulty following fast moving objects, tracking, fixating and scanning.	⊖ Prismatic glasses, eccentric viewing, some students may use one eye for distance tasks and one eye for near tasks.	✎ Close work may result in loss of place, eyestrain, blurring of print, poor concentration. Frequent rest periods may be needed when doing close work. Students may have difficulties in physical activities and may need more time to adjust to unfamiliar visual tasks. Classroom seating should favor the student's stronger eye.

Toxoplasmosis			
● Inflammation of the retina and choroid which causes scarring. Congenital toxoplasmosis infects the fetus in utero; acquired toxoplasmosis can develop anytime. ✛ Anti-inflammatory medications, photocoagulation, cryotheraphy. ▲ Caused by microorganisms found in animal feces and raw meat.	➠ Field loss, scotomas or blind spots, possibly loss of central vision, and squint. When the retinal damage is to the central area, see the adaptations and educational considerations in macular disease. When the damage is in the periphery, see the adaptations and educational considerations in retinitis pigmentosa.	✇ Microscopes, telescopes, eccentric viewing.	✎ High contrast line markers or templates may be helpful for reading, finding math problems or locating other important information.

Uveitis			
● Inflammation of the uveal tract which can involve the choroid, the ciliary body and or the iris. ▲ Can be caused by tuberculosis, histoplasmosis, toxoplasmosis.	➠ If the uveitis is acute or chronic anterior (iritis), there may be pain, photophobia and blurred vision. Other forms cause blurred vision, redness, and little or no pain.	✇ Good contrast and glare reduction, more time to adjust to new situations.	✎ Lights with rheostats and adjustable arms are helpful for close work.

Wilm's Tumor			
● Malignancy of the kidney, small stature, developmental delays. Often accompanies aniridia.	➠ Total or partial absence of iris, cataracts, ptosis, decreased visual acuity, photophobia, nystagmus.	✇ Pinhole contact lenses, tinted sunglasses and eye shades, dim lighting, rheostats, and lighting controls, magnification.	✎ Lighting conditions will need to be controlled to ensure optimal classroom performance. Teacher should not stand in front of window or light source when teaching or speaking to the student.

OTHER CONDITIONS THAT COULD HAVE IMPLICATIONS FOR THE EYE

Acquired immune deficiency syndrome (AIDS)

• A viral disease caused by the human immunodeficiency virus (HIV) which destroys the body's ability to fight infection. In the early stages symptoms include extreme fatigue, fever, night sweats, chills, swollen lymph glands, swollen spleen, loss of appetite, weight loss, severe diarrhea and depression. As the disease progresses, a form of pneumonia (pneumocystis carinii pneumonia) often occurs as wells as meningitis, encephalitis, tuberculosis, dementia, cytomegalovirus infection, and cancer (Karposis sarcoma). Many of these infections affect vision and may lead to total blindness.

Cytomegalovirus (CMV)

• A virus infection occurring congenitally and at any age. Symptoms are highly variable and may cause hemorrhaging, anemia, extensive liver or central nervous system damage. Chorioretinitis, microcephaly and cerebral calcification may also occur. Can cause hearing defects later.

Encephalitis

• An inflammation of the brain cells that is usually caused by a viral infection. Resulting conditions can include vision and speech disorders, difficulty in walking and personality changes. Recovery may be slow and death may result.

Meningitis

• An inflammation of the membranes that envelop the brain and spinal cord which can cause oculomotor palsies, ptosis, pupillary changes, photophobia and uveitis. Most commonly caused by bacterial infection.

Neurofibromatosis (von Recklinghausen's disease)

• A disease which is characterized by multiple benign tumors which appear anywhere in the body and light brown (café au lait) spots on the skin. There may be impairments to the bones, muscles and abdominal organs, and curvature of the spine can develop. Can cause papillidemia and optic atrophy.

Tumors

• An abnormal growth which can be benign or malignant and can affect any part of the visual system. While tumors of the eye are rare they are usually malignant and painless. See retinoblastoma for information about intraocular tumors.

Many students require prescription medication for their eye conditions. Here is a list of medications commonly prescribed with their purpose and possible side effects:

Ocular Medication	Eye Condition	Purpose	Side Effects ALERT PHYSICIAN!
Betagan	glaucoma	reduces production of fluid to lower pressure	unsteadiness, dizziness, confusion, headache, fatigue, troubled breathing, nausea
Dacriose	dryness of eye	irrigating solution	
Diamox	glaucoma	reduces production of fluid to lower pressure	
Enuclean Drops	prosthetic eyes: enucleation, anophthalmia	lubricant	
Ocutricin	conjunctivitis	antibiotic	itching, redness, swelling, rash
Pilocarpine	various ocular diseases and inflammation, glaucoma	constricts the pupil	few side effects noted
Propine	glaucoma	reduces production of fluid to lower pressure	fast or irregular heartbeat, increased blood pressure
Sodium Sulamyd	conjunctivitis, infections	antibiotic	itching, rash, swelling, redness
Timoptic	glaucoma	reduces production of fluid to lower pressure	anxiety, chest pain, confusion, diarrhea, headache, dizziness, stomach cramps, troubled breathing

Additional Readings and Resources

INFORMATION ABOUT THE EYE

Cassin, B. & Solomon, S. (1990). *Dictionary of eye terminology* (2nd ed.). Gainesville, FL: Triad.

Chalkney, T. (1982). *Your eyes* (2nd ed.). Springfield, IL: Charles Thomas.

Gregory, R. L. (1972). The eye. In *Eye and brain: The psychology of seeing.* New York: McGraw-Hill.

Jose, R. T. (Ed.). (1983). The eye and functional vision. In *Understanding low vision.* New York: American Foundation for the Blind.

Scholl, G. T. (Ed.) (1986). The visual system. In *Foundations of education for blind and visually handicapped children and youth: Theory and practice.* New York: American Foundation for the Blind.

Vaughan, D. & Ashbury, T. (1980). *General ophthalmology* (9th ed.). Los Altos, CA: Lang Medical.

Yeadon, A. & Grayson, D. (1979). How the eye works and eye disorders and diseases. In *Living with impaired vision: An introduction.* New York: American Foundation for the Blind.

DEVELOPMENTAL SEQUENCE OF VISION

Barraga, N. C. (1986). Sensory perceptual development. In G. T. Scholl (Ed.), *Foundations of education for blind and visually handicapped children and youth: Theory and practice.* New York: American Foundation for the Blind.

Barraga, N. C. & Collins, M. E. (1979). Development of efficiency in visual functioning: Rationale for a comprehensive program. *Journal of Visual Impairment and Blindness, 73,* 121-126.

Barraga, N. C. & Erin, J. N. (1992). Tactual, auditory, and visual development and learning. In *Visual handicaps and learning* (3rd ed.). Austin, TX: Pro•Ed.

Ferrell, K. (1987). Step-by-step charts in visual development. In L. Harrell & N. Akeson, *Preschool vision stimulation: It's more than a flashlight!* New York: American Foundation for the Blind.

Langley, M. B. (1980). Development of visual behaviors in the first three years of life. In *Functional vision inventory for the multiply and severely handicapped.* Chicago: Stoelting.

Barraga, N. C. & Morris, J. E. (1980). Major eye conditions and their influence on visual functioning. In *Program to develop efficiency in visual functioning: Source book on low vision.* Louisville, KY: American Printing House for the Blind.

Basso, L. V. (1987). The condition known as diabetes mellitus. *Journal of Visual Impairment and Blindness, 72,* 9, 338-342.

Bishop, V. E. (1986). *Selected anomalies and diseases of the eye.* Unpublished paper.

Cassin, B. & Solomon, S. (1990). *Dictionary of eye terminology* (2nd ed.). Gainesville, FL: Triad.

Coughlin, R. W. & Patz, A. (1978). Diabetic retinopathy: Nature and extent. *Journal of Visual Impairment and Blindness, 72,* 9, 343-347.

Duncan, E., Prickett, H. T., Finkelstein, D., Vernon, M., & Hollingsworth, T. (1988). *Usher's syndrome: What it is, how to cope, and how to help.* Springfield, IL: Charles Thomas.

Faye, E. E. (Ed.). (1984a). Case management of twenty-six common conditions. In *Clinical low vision* (2nd ed.). Boston: Little, Brown.

Faye, E. E. (Ed.). (1984b). The effect of the eye condition on functional vision. In *Clinical low vision* (2nd ed.). Boston: Little, Brown.

Gittenger, J. & Asdourian, G. (1988). *Manual of clinical problems in ophthalmology.* Boston: Little, Brown.

Glanze, W. D., Anderson, K. N., & Anderson, L. E. (1987). *The Signet/Mosby medical encyclopedia.* New York: C. V. Mosby.

Jan, J. E., Groenveld, M., & Sykanda, A. M. (1990). Light-gazing by visually impaired children. *Developmental Medicine and Child Neurology, 32,* 755-759.

Jan, J. E., Groenveld, M., Sykanda, A. M., & Hoyt, C. S. (1987). Behavioral characteristics of children with permanent cortical visual impairment. *Developmental Medicine and Child Neurology, 29,* 571-576.

Jose, R. T. (Ed.). (1983). The eye and functional vision. In *Understanding low vision.* New York: American Foundation for the Blind.

Kiester, E. (1990). *AIDS and vision loss.* New York: American Foundation for the Blind.

Nemshick, L. A., Vernon, M. C., & Ludman, F. (1986). The impact of retinitis pigmentosa on young adults: Psychological, educational, vocational and social considerations. *Journal of Visual Impairment and Blindness, 80,* 7, 859-862.

O'Dea, A. F. & Mayhall, C. A. (1988). Delayed manifestations of congenital rubella. *Journal of Visual Impairment and Blindness, 82,* 9, 379-381.

Pavan-Langston, D. (1985). *Manual of ocular diagnosis and therapy* (2nd ed.). Boston: Little, Brown.

Smith, A. J. & Cote, K. S. (1982). Common disorders and diseases of the eye. In *Look at me: A resource manual for the development of residual vision in multiply impaired children.* Philadelphia: Pennsylvania College of Optometry Press.

Tait, P. E. (1989). Optic nerve hypoplasia: A review of the literature. *Journal of Visual Impairment and Blindness, 83,* 4, 207-211.

Taylor, E. J., Anderson, D. M., Patwell, J. M., Plaut, K., & McCullough, K. (Eds.). (1988). *Dorland's illustrated medical dictionary* (27th ed.). Philadelphia: W. B. Saunders.

Trief, E., Duckman, R., Morse, A. R., & Silberman, R. K. (1989). Retinopathy of prematurity. *Journal of Visual Impairment and Blindness, 83,* 10, 500-504.

Upsal Low Vision Team. (n. d.). *Functional implications of diseases.* Unpublished paper.

Vernon, M. (n. d.). *Answers to your questions about Usher's syndrome.* Baltimore: National Retinitis Pigmentosa Foundation.

Yarkovishin, V. M. (1988). Coping with macular degeneration: From an optical perspective. *Journal of Visual Impairment and Blindness, 82,* 4, 127-128.

Yeadon, A. & Grayson, D. (1979). How the eye works and eye disorders and diseases. In *Living with impaired vision: An introduction.* New York: American Foundation for the Blind.

Zahn, J. R. (1989). Age-related maculopathy (ARM): The rehabilitative process. *Journal of Vision Rehabilitation, 3,* 1, 25-33.

Physical Conditions, the Sensory Systems, and How They Affect Visual Performance

by Gretchen Stone

There are a number of physical conditions and impairment to the sensory systems that influence visual performance. One would expect students who are multiply impaired or very young to demonstrate one or more of these physical limitations. However, to a lesser extent these same conditions can be found among older individuals who exhibit average or above average cognitive skills. These include:

- Changes in muscle tone
    - low muscle tone
    - increased muscle tone
    - fluctuating muscle tone

- Movement disorders
    - athetosis
    - spasticity
    - ataxia

- Reflex activity affecting posture
    - asymmetrical tonic neck reflex
    - symmetrical tonic neck reflex

- Postural control
    - poor balance
    - poor ocular-motor control
    - poor head control
    - poor sitting posture
    - muscle weakness

- Sensory impairments
    - Perception and the integration of vision with other forms of sensory input
    - Impairment of the tactile system
    - Inability to fully utilize vestibular sensation
    - Difficulty with depth perception
    - Difficulty with form perception
    - Difficulty perceiving the relative position of space

LOW MUSCLE TONE

When students experience low muscle tone their muscles are "floppy". Their muscles may actually feel soft to the touch. Individuals who have low muscle tone often look overweight even though they are not because their muscles are "sagging". Typically individuals with low muscle tone have poor posture. In some students low tone appears to be related to a decrease in deep sensory input (proprioceptive and vestibular input), although direct cause and effect have not been established. It is known that visual, tactile, and auditory stimulation can affect levels of awareness which in turn influence posture and balance.

Low muscle tone is a neurological problem that is present at birth. The condition is frequently referred to as hypotonia. It is a very common problem among individuals who experience multiple impairments, especially Down's syndrome. Students with low tone may have excessive range of motion in their joints, particularly in the shoulders and hips. Proper positioning is essential. Proper positioning influences tone and thus enhances the functional capacity of students.

Low muscle tone may not appear to be related to visual performance, but low tone can influence how well students are able to direct their gaze. Neck extension and head control have far reaching effects throughout the entire trunk. Students with low tone position their heads so that they have optimal control over their entire bodies. Head positioning that facilitates trunk support may be in conflict with head positioning that directs gaze. Following are some examples of how low tone can influence visual performance and how programming can be adapted to compensate for underlying problems:

Programming for Compensation

- Situation #1:
  A child may be trying to put on his shoes when seated in a chair, but he neglects to look at his feet. Instead he looks up at the ceiling. Although it seems reasonable to ask him to watch what he is doing, maintaining a sitting posture while reaching down to his feet may be so difficult that if he looks down he may fall out of the chair. In fact, the child is hyperextending his neck, that is, he is using a primitive reflex pattern to maintain his posture in the chair.

  An alternative approach to this task would be to place the student on the floor in the corner of the room where he can use both sides of the wall for support and reach his feet without fear of falling.

- Situation #2:
  A student who has low tone may be reluctant to move freely about the environment. This may interfere with orientation and mobility training. She feels at risk because she has difficulty returning to a stable position when her balance is threatened. When her vision limits her ability to anticipate potential obstacles, she feels even more vulnerable. Delayed equilibrium reactions may compound the problem. If equilibrium reactions are delayed she may not be able to respond quickly enough to situations that upset her balance, she may be more prone to falling or injuring herself.

  When she is moving throughout her environment, be certain she has the muscular control to move over uneven terrain without support. Give her warnings that she is approaching a challenging situation. Give her a stabilizing assist at one elbow if she is in potential danger.

- Situation #3:
  A student may be sitting in a chair while manipulating an object. Slowly she starts to slump to one side or the other. Because she does not return her head to the midline of her body, her eyes begin to wander away from the task. Her attention begins to wane.

  To prevent this, when a student with low tone is performing manipulative tasks, make sure that she is properly seated, with her feet flat on the floor. Her forearms should rest on the table surface. In this way she uses her arms to stabilize her trunk. If she is asked to use her hands without support she may slump to one side or the other. She may be able to lift her arms to manipulate objects, but the conscious effort of manipulating the object and maintaining her posture in the chair may reduce her attention span. She may also have difficulty stabilizing movements that are initiated from the shoulder. This makes it all the more difficult for her to use her hands and to perform fine motor activities.

  In this situation, as in most others, the teacher must consider programming goals. If the goal is to increase sitting tolerance and to work on increasing muscle control while sitting, then the manipulative task becomes secondary. If, however, the task itself is being targeted, then providing external means of support would be justified. Support could include side supports for the chair or hip (lateral) support as suggested by an occupational therapist or physical therapist.

  Students who are hypotonic are especially susceptible to subluxation at the shoulder girdle. (This means that the muscles do not hold the bones in position in the shoulder area.)
  It is very important never to lift students by the arms to shift their sitting posture or to pull them to standing by grabbing their arms.

- Situation #4:

  A student is looking up toward the ceiling or sky in search of a light source. He is not directing his gaze to the task at hand.

  Direct the student's gaze by pointing from his eyes to the direction of the targeted object, or by gently but firmly moving his head. Whether he is sitting or standing, it is important to refrain from pushing his head down abruptly. In doing so, you are likely to influence overall tone. You may trigger a flexor pattern that would make it more difficult to perform the task.

Note:

A student who has extremely low muscle tone may direct his attention toward maintaining postural control in a sitting position. This may detract from visual performance.

Students who experience extremely low muscle tone usually benefit from the services of occupational and/or physical therapists. In many cases positioning, seating systems, and other adaptive equipment are needed. Therapeutic intervention is most effective when instructional personal, therapists, and family members work together to come up with the best solutions for the students' needs in a variety of situations. Physical and occupational therapists can be a resource in helping teachers make distinctions between activities that students cannot do because of their visual limitations, as opposed to the ones they cannot do because of problems with muscle tone.

Note:

Students who are cortically visually impaired (CVI) exhibit different response patterns than typically found among students with poor visual acuity. Cortically visually impaired children may turn their heads to get a visual fix on objects using their peripheral vision. Also, when doing some motor tasks they may look away from the task by turning their head to the side and looking downward.

INCREASED MUSCLE TONE

Many students who experience multiple handicapping conditions develop increased muscle tone or hypertonicity.

By itself, increased muscle tone may not appear to influence vision, but increased muscle tone can influence how well students are able to direct their gaze. Students who are unable to move freely often cannot orient themselves to the source of visual stimulation. They must hold their bodies in a rigid posture. Visual stimulation can trigger increased muscle tone. Students who are hypertonic are often hyper-reactive to visual input. Following are some examples of situations in which increased muscle tone affects vision:

- A student is sitting in a chair and someone enters the room. He is unable to turn and look at the person.

- An object is moving across the room. The student's ability to track the object is limited because she cannot move her head without triggering increased tone throughout her body.

Programming for Compensation

Students who have increased muscle tone may not be able to function optimally in a sitting position. Sitting requires a considerable amount of control. In order to facilitate visual performance it may be helpful to try working with students in a supine or sidelying position.

Each of these examples requires the services of occupational and physical therapists who can offer child-specific suggestions. In many cases positioning, seating systems, and other adaptive equipment are needed. Therapeutic intervention is most effective when instructional personnel, therapists, and family members work together to come up with the best solutions for the students' needs in a variety of situations.

Fluctuating muscle tone is often associated with athetosis and severe seizure disorders. Tone usually changes from hypotonic to hypertonic. Individuals with fluctuating tone have a limited ability to hold postures needed for control of limb movement. Following is a situation that might be expected of a student who experiences fluctuations in muscle tone:

- The student may appear relaxed when lying on the floor, but when she is moved to a sitting position for mealtime she may tighten her muscles and become rigid. The process of eating or even visual stimulation may be enough to trigger a change in tone.

Again, students who exhibit these problems require the services of occupational and physical therapists. In many cases positioning, seating systems, and other adaptive equipment are needed. Therapeutic intervention is most effective when instructional personnel, therapists, and family members work together to come up with the best solutions for the students' needs in a variety of situations.

FLUCTUATING MUSCLE TONE

Programming for Compensation

Movement Disorders

ATHETOSIS

The most common movement disorder is athetosis. Students who experience athetosis move their limbs or head slowly, involuntarily, and constantly. There is usually severe involvement in the hands. In one form of athetosis the individual is forced into patterns of extension.

SPASTICITY

Spasticity results in muscle imbalances, contractures, and sometimes deformities in the bones. Spasticity limits the number of postures students can assume, and it makes weightshifting more difficult. Some surgical procedures are available that reduce spasticity in some areas of the body.

- A student chronically maintains a flexed position. His neck is down while his arms and legs are tightly held in a fixed position. He stares into his own lap and does not gain information about events around him.

- A student chronically maintains an extended position. Her head is extended back and she is reclined in the chair so that she is looking at the ceiling.

- A student is unable to maintain his posture unsupported without conscious effort unless he is positioned in a sidelying position on a mat. Sitting in a chair or standing at a standing table is exhausting. His perspective of the environment is distorted and he has difficulty orienting himself to changes in the environment.

- Due to chronically contracted muscles, a student cannot move her arms or legs through a full range of motion. Consequently the student is limited in her ability to move around in the environment or to manipulate toys, or to perform other functional activities.

Another movement disorder is ataxia. Students who experience ataxia are unable to coordinate their muscles, and they may be unable to walk. Many students who exhibit ataxia are able to walk with walkers and/or crutches. Those who can walk independently may demonstrate a wide-based, swaying gait. Sample situations that might be expected of students who experience movement disorders are:

* Situation #1:
  A student is positioned in an adapted seat. His head is constantly turning from side to side. He is unable to control his gaze, nor can he control his hands enough to move objects within his visual field. He may have adequate vision, but his lack of head control makes it impossible for him to use it.

* Situation #2:
  Walking is so difficult for a student that all her attention is focused on remaining upright. Concern for watching where she is going is secondary.

Each of these disorders requires the services of occupational and physical therapists. In many cases positioning, seating systems, and other adaptive equipment are needed. Therapeutic intervention is most effective when instructional personal, therapists, and family members work together to come up with the best solutions for the student's needs in a variety of situations. A VH teacher needs to determine which activities the students cannot do because of their visual limitations as opposed to the ones they cannot do because of problems with tone, and consult with a therapist.

ATAXIA

PROGRAMMING
FOR
COMPENSATION

Reflex Activity Affecting Posture

Postural reflexes are normally present in infancy, but as students mature most reflexes are integrated into the central nervous system so that individuals can develop voluntary control over their own movements. As these reflexes become integrated, they provide a postural base for controlled movement. Most reflexes are integrated by the time infants are six months old. The following reflexes influence postural control:

ASYMMETRICAL TONIC NECK REFLEX (ATNR)

This reflex is activated by moving the head to one side. When the head turns to one side, the arm and leg on the side of the body toward the face side extend, and the arm and leg on the skull side of the body are flexed. In infancy this reflex is useful because it stimulates visually guided reaching. However, when this reflex is not fully integrated it may interfere with feeding, midline use of the hands, and body symmetry. Even though it appears that a student has integrated this reflex, the ATNR may be elicited when the student is exerting a great deal of effort on a particularly difficult task. Presenting materials at midline decreases the likelihood that this reflex will be elicited.

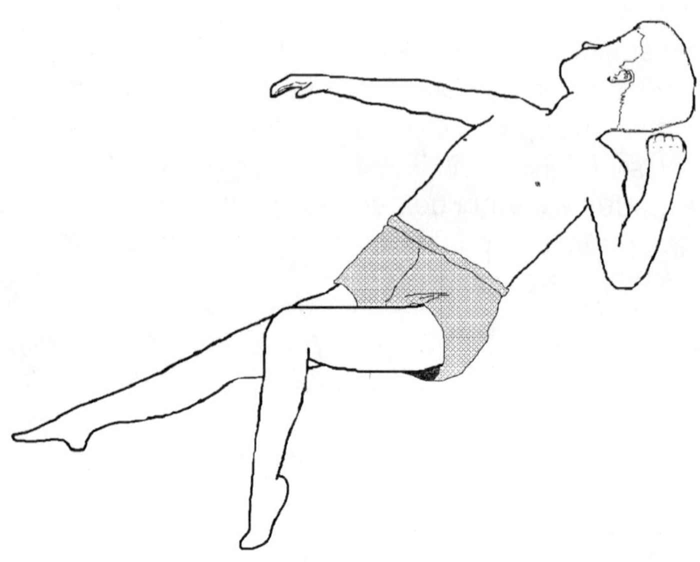

This is activated when the neck is flexed or extended. When the neck is extended, the arms extend and the legs flex. When the neck is flexed, the arms flex and the legs extend. When the student is lying on her stomach this reflex interferes with her ability to weight-bear on her arms. It also interferes with creeping and crawling. In sitting, the STNR interferes with functional use of the arms and hands on a tray or table. For example, if the student raises her head to look up, the arms straighten, pushing her hands away from the activity. Extending the legs during neck flexion may cause the student to thrust out of the chair.

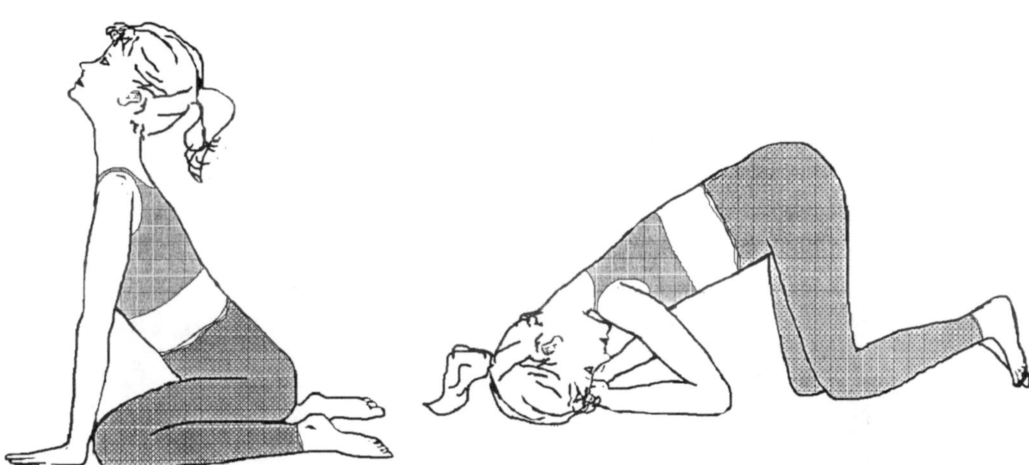

Although occupational and physical therapists work with students to help integrate these reflexes, instructional personnel and family members can develop a keen sense of awareness of when a reflex is interfering with visually oriented activities. Service providers who are unaware of the influence of reflexes may interpret the students actions as avoidance behaviors rather than involuntary responses. For example, students may appear to look directly at an object and then intentionally push it away, when in reality they are unable to control arm extension when their head is turned. Students may flex their neck to look down at an object that is positioned close to their body, which in turn causes them to push out of the chair. This could be misinterpreted as an attempt to get out of the chair. Close communication with therapists can help define practices that minimize reflexive actions, and to interpret situations in which they do occur.

Postural Control

POOR BALANCE

Optical righting reactions are patterns of movement in which vision stimulates the head to rise to a normal position. This means that even when the body is held in a nonvertical position, students are able to move their heads so that their face is vertical to the floor and their mouth is horizontal to the floor. Thus, students are able to hold their head upright even when their bodies are tilted.

Equilibrium reactions enable students to move around without losing their balance. They help students to recognize a change in the center of gravity and to move their bodies accordingly. Equilibrium reactions trigger a coordinated motor response that will help students to constantly change their body alignment.

When individuals who experience multiple impairments have difficulty with balance it is almost always due to immature or ineffective equilibrium and righting reactions. Students use righting reactions to get into and maintain an upright position for walking. Righting reactions are also used to return the body to the normal position in space when balance has been challenged or to adjust parts of the body to a vertical position. The righting reactions depend upon visual information and vestibular input.

There is some evidence to suggest that the cerebellum or "balance center" of the brain influences control of eye movements. Therefore, students who experience cerebellar dysfunction may also experience difficulties with ocular-motor control.

Sample situations that might be expected of students who experience problems with optical righting reactions and equilibrium reactions:

• Situation #1:
  When a student does not have adequately developed righting reactions, she does not automatically orient her head and trunk in space and to the ground. She may hold her head to one side or the other or sway her head from side to side in search of vestibular stimulation. She may walk by side stepping, shifting her weight laterally from one leg to the other in an awkward fashion. She may have difficulty maintaining balance on one leg while stepping forward with the other. This is often very noticeable in stair climbing and she may want to ascent sideways holding two hands on the rail.

• Situation #2:
  A student may be threatened by movement across an uneven surface. He has no assurance that he will regain his balance if he starts to fall. He fears that he will injure himself.

• Situation #3:
  A student hangs off a piece of playground or play equipment or hangs off the side of a bed without attempting to return to a position of stability. She may lose postural control or balance when walking assisted. It is important to observe if she is using a cane or pre-cane device for support instead of as an orientation and mobility tool. It is also important to evaluate her sighted guide technique.

Note:
It is possible to develop equilibrium and righting reactions through adulthood if therapeutic intervention is provided.

POOR OCULAR-MOTOR CONTROL

Ocular-motor control includes ocular fixation on stationary objects and ocular pursuit (180 degrees). The muscles involved in extra-ocular control are influenced by the vestibulo-ocular reflexes. These reflexes are strongly influenced by the vestibular system which detects the body's response to gravity and movement through space. The vestibular nerve terminates in the semi-circular canals near the ears. Each time the head moves, one or more of the semicircular canals are stimulated, and each time they are stimulated, one or more pairs of the six pairs of muscles that move the eyeball are affected. Stimulation of the semicircular canals also affects muscles in the arms, legs, and neck.

The optical righting reflex helps keep the body upright. The role of this reflex becomes obvious when students' standing balance with eyes open is compared with their standing balance with eyes closed.

In addition to the optical righting reflex, ocular movement is believed to have an effect on some of the postural reflexes including the righting reactions. There is some evidence that looking to the side can trigger neck righting reactions and possibly the tonic neck reflex.

This close interrelationship between eye musculature and postural reactions provides the theoretical basis for sensory integrative therapy. It is thought that activating and normalizing postural mechanisms, especially on the stomach and in all fours positions, helps to improve extra-ocular muscle control. The rationale is that sensorimotor integration activities will encourage the eye musculature to perform in a normal manner. Poor ocular-motor control affects performance on a wide variety of academic tasks. These tasks include handwriting, copying from the chalkboard, reading, and following sequences of numbers and letters.

Programming for Compensation

A sensory integrative treatment program for normalizing postural mechanisms would be initiated by an occupational therapist or physical therapist. Some programming activities can be carried out by parents or by other members of the student's instructional team.

In addition to maintaining a vertical position in space, head control involves:

(1) controlled rotation of the head,
(2) controlled movements from side to side, and
(3) lifting the head while laying on back or stomach.

Neck rotation activates the rest of the body to turn in the same direction as the face so that the head and trunk are aligned with each other. When the head is turned to the right nearly to the shoulder (ATNR), extensor tone is increased on the right and flexor tone is increased on the left. The reverse is true when the head is turned to the left. When the head is prone (i. e., lying on the stomach), flexor muscles are facilitated. When the head is supine (i. e., lying on the back), extensor muscles are facilitated. Examples of poor head control include:

• A student may be unable to use his arms or hands while he is lying on his stomach. He cannot support his weight or lift his head.

• A student is lying on her back. She is able to look at midline but she arches her back, and her legs extend if she moves her head away from midline.

Position students on their stomach at the end of a large wedge while providing support at the shoulders. Let their arms and hands fall to the floor surface and provide materials for manipulation on a surface below the body to counteract the effects of working against gravity. In this position students are able to watch their hands as they manipulate objects.

Position students on their back and suspend objects at midline for them to manipulate. Encourage bilateral use of arms and hands.

Note:
Upright positions are more likely to facilitate an alerting response. Occupational or physical therapists can offer positioning suggestions and equipment to provide support when head control is poor.

POOR HEAD CONTROL

Programming for Compensation

POOR SITTING POSTURE

Orientation of the head and sitting posture influence ocular-motor control. Examples of poor sitting positions include:

- A student slumps to one side or the other.

- A student bends forward in her seat.

- A student thrusts forward in the seat.

Programming for Compensation

Whenever students are poorly positioned it effects their ability to use their vision. Poor sitting posture is a manifestation of nearly all of the other problems listed in this section. These include: low muscle tone, increased muscle tone, movement disorders, changes in muscle tone, reflex activity that affects posture, poor balance, poor head control, and muscle weakness.

Students who exhibit these problems require the services of occupational and physical therapists. In many cases positioning, seating systems, and other adaptive equipment are needed. For optimal benefit, all those working with these students need to be consistent in using good positioning practices. This consistency is vital to the prevention of future skeletal deformities.

Muscle weakness is lack of strength in the muscles. A student who is visually impaired may develop muscle weakness because she is less physically active than her sighted peers. If this is extreme, poor muscle strength can affect the ability to maintain static postures (e. g., sitting, standing) as well as any movements through space. Muscle weakness can make it difficult for her to move from a lying to sitting position or from a sitting position to a standing position unaided. Muscle weakness affects her orientation and mobility skills.

Students who experience visual impairment often develop different patterns of muscle use and may engage in fewer activities that require resistive movement patterns. They may be less likely to integrate proprioceptive information because of lack of visual feedback that usually accompanies movement through space. Therefore, movement tends to be less meaningful.

Many students who are visually impaired and also multiply impaired do not enjoy rigorous activity. The reasons may include poor tone, poor equilibrium and righting reactions and the lack of social rewards. Regular exercise programs are essential for these students. Depending on the extent of the students' physical impairment, the occupational therapist and/or physical therapist should be involved in developing and monitoring appropriate physical activities which can be carried out by family members and school staff.

MUSCLE
WEAKNESS

Programming for
Compensation

The Sensory Systems

Sometimes the sensory systems are divided into two categories: the near senses (touch, movement, taste, and smell) and the far senses (vision and hearing). Although all of the sensory systems work together, they each have a unique contribution to make. The seven sensory systems are:

- **Gustation and olfaction**
  This is commonly known as taste and smell.

- **Visceral sensation**
  The visceral receptors are located in the body's internal organs. They provide information by responding to stretch. For example, people know to stop eating when their stomach is stretched, that is, they feel full.

- **Audition**
  This is commonly known as hearing

- **Vision**
  This is commonly known as sight.

- **Touch**
  The sensation of touch includes sensitivity to light touch, pressure, pain, and temperature.

- **Proprioception**
  The proprioceptors are receptors in joints, muscles, tendon, and fascia. They provide information about the relative positions of parts of the body and provide feedback after motor action.

- **Vestibular sensation**
  Receptors in the inner ear provide information about movement. Different vestibular receptors are sensitive to rotary and linear acceleration in space (e. g., movement in circles or in a straight line) and to displacement of the head in relation to gravity.

Although the first three sensory systems (gustation and olfaction, visceral and audition) are integrated with the visual system, they do not have as many implications for programming as do the following three sensory systems (tactile, proprioceptive, and vestibular).

"It is the integration of the sensory systems that causes development and development which facilitates further integration" (Banus, 1971). If the sensory systems "cause" development, then assessment designed to evaluate sensory processing should focus on the **quality** of student's responses and should seek to determine **why** students react as they do. Observing student's reactions to sensory information will lead to awareness about whether they are hypo- or hyper-reactive to different forms of sensory input. Ongoing assessment will lead to understanding as to why students react in certain ways in specific situations. For example, if a student is highly agitated in the school cafeteria it may be assumed that his behavior is related to eating, when, in fact, he is reacting to the noise in the cafeteria. He may have a heightened sensitivity to auditory input.

The purpose of sensory programming is to enable students to use sensory input and to structure the environment so that students will be motivated to explore the environment and to find meaning in the world. Sensory programming is more likely to be effective when students are actively initiating responses rather than passively receiving sensory input.

Sensory input is the most basic way that students receive information from the surrounding environment. Sensory input is organized by the central nervous system and the peripheral nervous system in ways that enable students to discover things that occur around them.

Sensory input or sensation is closely related to arousal. Arousal increases the likelihood that students will orient themselves to a new source of stimulation. When students orient to a stimulus, their heads typically move in the direction of the stimulus, and various physiological changes occur. These physiological changes help students to be more receptive to the stimulus. They also help students to create a state of readiness in case it becomes necessary for them to take action. When the processing of visual input is impaired, this orienting response is altered because turning the head to the source of the stimulus gives little or no visual information. Students become less likely to orient their heads to new stimulation. Because of the way in which the head and neck influence the overall tone of the whole body, students with visual impairments may have a diminished state of readiness for reaching out in the environment.

In part, the positions of the head and neck are able to influence the tone of the whole body because, like other parts of the body, they have sensory receptors. Some sensory input originates from receptors in the joints, and tissues of the body. Other sensory input originates from the environment and is received by sensory receptors in the body. Overall, the body is organized so that sensory input is paired with motor output. After receiving, processing, and evaluating input, students have the opportunity to take an active role in the world through motor output. This becomes cyclical in that every time students move they get additional sensory feedback. This gives them new opportunities for assessing the environment. Active participation in this sensory-motor process can greatly influence later learning.

Perception helps students to make sense out of the potentially over-whelming number and variety of sensations that they receive at any given time. Perceptual processes organize or integrate sensations into mean-ingful chunks of information. Often the term perceptual "development" is used because it is known that when students have past experiences with sensation, it easier for them to integrate new sensations. Perception is a developing process.

Sometimes perceptual development is altered because the brain fails to process information from the eyes. Students may have problems with "central processing" of visual information. The structures which transmit visual information to the brain are intact, but the information reaching the brain is not processed or interpreted in a meaningful way. An extreme example of this is cortical visual impairment. As stated earlier, cortical visual impairment may be considered to be a sensory processing or perceptual problem rather than a problem with "vision" or visual sensory input.

Note:
It is often difficult to draw the line between the input of information (sensation) and the processing of information (perception). One distinc-tion is that perception involves the simultaneous processing of more than one sensation. This applies to sensations arising from the same sensory system or from sensations arising from more than one sensory system. Another distinction is that perception involves processing, whereas sensation traditionally refers just to the reception of information.

HOW PERCEPTION
INTEGRATES
SENSORY INPUT

"Tactile sensitivity or awareness refers to the ability to receive and interpret stimuli through contact with the skin and exploration with the hands. Through the manipulation of objects, a child develops discriminations of temperature, texture, hardness or contour. When such tactile contact is meaningful, it can be integrated with information he gains visually and by audition, giving a richer and more pleasurable experience. When tactile contact is disturbing or not meaningful, there is a tendency to withdraw from or avoid such contact with the environment." (Banus, 1971, p. 290).

Tactile discrimination becomes more important when students have little or no visual input. Exploration through touch becomes a primary source of gaining information about the environment. The tactile system is often thought of as two separate systems: one is a discriminative system that helps students to identify objects in the environment; the other is a protective system that helps students to detect objects or situations in the environment that are potentially threatening.

Students who experience multiple impairments often demonstrate neurological damage. Because the tactile system is so extensive and because it interacts with so many of the other sensory systems, damage to the nervous system as a whole often involves damage to the tactile system.

Examples of how the tactile systems and vision are related and how programming can be adapted to compensate for the underlying problem include:

- *Students consider light touch to be aversive, that is, they are tactually defensive.*

  Some students delight in rough play and they like massages, body pounding, and rough textures, but they are unable to tolerate light touch. Areas that are particularly sensitive are those around their lips, the palms of their hands, and the soles of their feet. When students are very sensitive in these areas they may hate to have their faces washed, their socks put on, walking in bare feet, touching soft and fuzzy toys. On the other hand they may particularly enjoy vibration, cold objects such as ice cubes, and rough textures such as sand paper.

  When children are overly sensitive to light touch, the part of the tactile system that has a protective function is overriding the part of the tactile system that has a discriminative function. Students need to have "tactile success" to diminish their fight or flight reaction, which is a protective function. Although tactile defensiveness is less likely to occur when students are actively engaged in activity rather than receiving stimulation passively, aversion to some textures may interfere with everyday activities such as asking them to wipe the toothpaste from their mouths.

  Water activities are sometimes effective in helping students to overcome their reluctance to explore and manipulate objects with their hands. Because the feel of water is pleasant to most students, they may be more likely to poke at objects, retrieve objects, and later manipulate them without encountering unpleasant experiences. Ice cubes can be added to lukewarm water for contrasts in temperature.

  Additional activities can be designed to offer some resistance to actively manipulating materials that are presented. Students can find objects hidden in sand. Then students can move from work with mud and soft dough to clay. They can be encouraged to push, pull, roll, squeeze, and poke the material. Emphasis is not on producing some specific finished product, but on experimental manipulation.

- *Students have reduced perceptions of pain.*

  This can be particularly dangerous for individuals who experience visual impairments because they may encounter objects or events that are harmful, but their withdrawal from these events may be delayed. It is not uncommon for students who are multiply involved to suffer a burn from a toaster, to sustain a bite from a peer, to pick or rub a sore on their bodies until it bleeds, or to get a bruise and yet not cry out or show distress in any way. Students may get hurt and caregivers may not be able to explain how or when the injury occurred. Whenever possible, model language for them by naming the injured body part and giving a simple explanation of cause and effect.

  Little can be done to eliminate the cause of this problem, but all instructional staff and caregivers need to be aware of the problem and to take additional measures to protect their students from potential hazardous situations.

- *Students are unable to localize tactile stimuli.*

  Sometimes students may not be sure of what touched them or they may not be able to locate where they were touched. If they are touched in two places at the same time, they may be aware of being touched in one place, but not the other. This interferes with students' orientation to the environment in general. It also interferes with their ability to defend themselves from potentially dangerous encounters in the environment.

  Sometimes students can increase their ability to localize tactile stimuli by participating in activities such as removing rolled pieces of masking tape from different parts of their bodies, playing imitation games where they co-actively rub a part of their bodies that an instructor has previously touched. Whenever possible, these activities should be infused into functional activities. Occupational therapists should be able to provide a wide range of activities in this area.

- *Students may continue to mouth materials past ages when this is developmentally appropriate.*

While mouthing past the second year of life is generally not appropriate for sighted children, mouthing is often very functional for students who are unable to use their vision to discriminate among the properties of objects. Babies learn to mouth before they are able to use their hands. Developmentally, mouthing toys and different textures contributes to the students' tolerance of foods with different textures. They discontinue mouthing as they develop visual discrimination and manual manipulation skills. When students are not able to use their vision to discriminate, they are likely to engage in mouthing activities for a longer period of time. This problem is compounded by the subsequent lack of experiences that encourage the development of manipulative skills. Students will often use their mouth to stabilize an object as they adjust their hand grasp. This tends to limit development in hand-manipulative skills. When students experience visual impairments they are less likely to encounter objects in the environment or to notice features of objects that offer potentially new information through manipulation.

Sometimes students will just touch objects to their faces, often near the lips, and then they will manipulate these objects with their hands. This behavior becomes functional because it helps them to identify objects. It may be appropriate in some situations. However, when touching objects to the face becomes habitual, it becomes problematic. For example, students may handle eating utensils or objects that are used by other people. In general, it is best to discourage mouthing and to introduce objects that offer interesting information as they are being manipulated.

- *Students have a diminished alerting system and do not respond to their environment unless contact is intense.*

  Students who do not seek tactile input, because it does not appear to be meaningful, frequently have delays in sensory-motor development. They do not explore, therefore they do not learn about the environment. It is essential for these students to become actively involved in a broad range of activities, even though they may not be self-initiated.

  It is often helpful to raise the overall level of arousal of these students by rough housing, vigorous rocking, body rubbing or vibrations before attempting to engage them in purposeful activity. Students who are "hyperreactive" or under-reactive to stimulation are at risk because it is often easy to ignore them. They are likely to sit or lay quietly, causing few problems. They may sleep a lot or they may complain loudly if aroused. It may be necessary for instructional staff to be sure to set regularly scheduled times to interact with students who have these needs so they are not forgotten in a classroom filled with more demanding students.

Proprioception refers to information arising from the body, especially from muscles, joints, ligaments, and receptors associated with bones. Students usually become aware of these sensations only when they deliberately focus their attention on them. The proprioceptors are a critical part of three kinds of movement, including reflexes, automatic responses, and planned actions. These kinds of movements help students to adapt themselves to and act upon the environment.

The proprioceptors help to integrate sensory input through motor actions. They aid in sensory perception, especially perception of visual information. In turn, vision plays an important role in awareness of joint position and skilled motor movements. Students are able to know when their arms are up or down or are bent or extended, by feeling these positional changes without any visual clues. However, it is this internal process of feeling motor movements, in combination with visual feedback, that allows students to monitor or refine patterns of movement. Students without visual impairments are able to watch their movements. They learn to use their vision to correct and refine their movements. Therefore, vision is closely related to kinesthesia, the conscious awareness of joint position and movement.

When students are not aware of joint position and movement, this limits their development of visual perception and their body scheme by limiting the amount of information entering the brain during purposeful and manipulative tasks. In addition, proprioceptors in the extraocular muscles of the eyes appear to provide information about visual form and space perception.

Thus, proprioceptive and tactile input helps students to perceive spatial relationships. Students use this processing to develop a stable visual field and to be able to use information about the environment from different points of view. This enables them to develop an awareness of their motor capabilities at any given point in space and time.

Probably the most obvious example of proprioceptive loss is demonstrated by students who have experienced a stroke on one side of the body. Although these students may be able to walk, as they take a step they do not know where to place their foot without looking. Injuries are common as students with this problem bear their weight on a turned ankle or let their foot drop from the footrest of a wheelchair so that it drags or gets caught on something.

Other examples are students who have difficulty performing simple gymnastic stunts, or are unable to follow a path. They may not be able to figure out how to push or pull a wagon or to guide their movements as they walk through a crowded place. It may be difficult for them to use riding toys or to play simple games that require them to coordinate their movements with other students. Carrying a tray in the cafeteria may be especially difficult as they try to manage both upper and lower extremities. They may overreach or underreach for objects. In general, students who experience proprioceptive loss may be thought to be clumsy.

Sometimes students are unable to maintain cane positions or other arm positions during orientation and mobility activities because they do not receive sufficient feedback from the proprioceptive system to allow them to maintain fixed positions in space.

To help students become more aware of the position and movement of their arms and hands, apply resistance to their movements. Activities may include pushing a heavy object (such as a two-pound sandbag) across the table as far as they can with two hands and then pull it back. Instructional staff can play push/pull body games, or if the student is older, tug of war while sitting in a chair. Contrast this with pushing and pulling light objects and then pushing and pulling using only one hand. This activity can be varied even further by pushing a heavy object with one hand and a light object with another and trying to keep them even.

Students can lift a heavy object on one side and a light object on the other. They can place weighted objects into containers at varying distances. Students can imitate a limb position on one side to match a position in which they have been placed on the opposite side.

Occupational and physical therapists should be a valuable resource in helping to design activities that stimulate proprioceptive awareness. These activities can be incorporated into regular educational programming. Songs and body movements associated with a rhythm can be helpful to establish some success with motor planning. Auditory cues can help to monitor movement. Students may need to be taught strategies for activities such as riding toys or positioning themselves in a chair.

PROGRAMMING
FOR
COMPENSATION

The vestibular system enables students to detect motion, especially acceleration and deceleration and the earth's gravitational pull. The system helps students to know whether any form of sensory input (i. e., visual, tactile, or proprioceptive) is associated with movement of the body or is only evident in the external environment.

Vestibular sensation is closely related to visual orientation through a feedback loop. Based on both vestibular input and visual input, the body is able to restore itself to a given orientation or equilibrium position when disturbed. These systems help the body to maintain stability.

The simplest behavioral response to disturbed orientation is the righting reflex. The righting reflex can be elicited when the body receives information from the visual system indicating that the head is no longer vertical. When vision is not present this feedback is still provided from the vestibular system. When the head is tilted to one side, the fluid in the semicircular canals moves around. The vestibular nerve is sensitive to the movement of fluid in the semicircular canals and signals the need for the extraocular muscles to rotate the eye about the visual axis when the head is tilted to the side. This is done on a reflexive basis. Thus, the vestibular system and the visual system work together, but when the visual system is not operating, the vestibular system can partially compensate for lack of visual input.

Sighted students will show nystagmus following spinning activities. This illustrates the close connection between the vestibular system and the extraocular muscles of the eye. Since many students with visual impairments have a resting nystagmus, this response is not always a good indication of vestibular functioning among this special population.

Examples of how vestibular sensation and vision are related and how programming can be adapted to compensate for underlying problems include:

* *Students become very calm or act disturbed when they are riding in cars or other vehicles.*

  The processing of vestibular sensation tells students whether they are moving within a room or whether it is the room that is moving. Are they moving in a car, or is it the car that is moving? Is this school bus going slow or fast? Has this school bus just gone over a speed bump? Through the vestibular system student gain information about the world that is not available to them through vision.

  Some students who are agitated become calm when riding in a car. The rhythmic ride as well as the sudden stops and starts provide an optimal level of arousal. Other students become very agitated as they sense a loss of control while they are moving through space. For these students, very slow rides in parking lots may be a beginning activity. Sitting close to a caregiver may provide enough support to dispel perceptions of being vulnerable. Tightened seatbelts provide additional security.

* *Students fail to increase their muscle tone in response to movement through space.*

  Vestibular stimulation has a strong influence on muscle tone. This is true of overall tone, but also in terms of certain neuromuscular reflexes. For example, as students lie prone on a scooterboard and move down a ramp, an increase in extensor tone can be expected as the vestibular input stimulates muscles responsible for extending the trunk and neck. Sighted students would take note of the incline and prepare by extending their trunk and head to avoid falling off the scooterboard or hitting their head along the ride down the incline.

  Although the response is likely to be delayed, students who are visually impaired still elicit their extensor muscles in response to vestibular input. There are many and varied activities for accomplishing this reaction. This is an area of expertise that is common among occupational and physical therapists. They may suggest programming activities that can be implemented by others who work with students.

- *Students who are visually impaired often engage in stereotypic or repetitive behaviors that provide them with vestibular input.*

  Swinging on a swing or swaying back and forth in a chair are ways of gaining vestibular stimulation. Sometimes members of the instructional team allow students to sway in a chair or swing for long periods of time, using the rationale that this type of stimulation is "good for them." This is not a solid rationale because only the starting and the stopping of the motion elicits adaptive vestibular responses. Vestibular adaptation occurs during acceleration and deceleration, not during prolonged, rhythmic activity. Rhythmic activity may be calming, but is does not elicit adaptive responses, therefore it does not contribute to development or to increased functional skills.

  Many self-stimulatory activities may be closely related to the reticular activating system as well as to the vestibular system. This is because the vestibular system and the reticular activating system are related to one another. The reticular activating system monitors levels of alertness and attention. Swaying activities may become rhythmic and can serve as a means of either reducing or eliciting stimulation. Such activities are body oriented, and internally focused. Because they serve to isolate students from the outside world, self-stimulatory activities interfere with new learning.

  In other words, many self-stimulating activities serve to depress brain activity rather than to stimulate brain activity. Focus of attention is not on meaningful stimuli.

- *Students appear to be hypo-reactive to vestibular stimulation.*

  These students do not show a noticeable change in nystagmus and do not appear to become dizzy following spinning activities. Often these students seem to crave vestibular-based activity when young, but as they become older they can no longer tolerate the same level of intensity. In general, child initiated activity that results in vestibular input should be encouraged as long as it does not take the form of stereotypic behavior.

- *Students change their tolerance for movement activities over time.*

  Many young children with visual impairments seem to have a nearly endless toleration for merry-go-rounds, spinning in tire swings, and swaying or swinging on other playground equipment. However, the need for intense vestibular stimulation seems to be age-related. During and following adolescence, students who previously seemed to have a nearly insatiable need for vestibular stimulation lower their tolerance for vestibular-related activities. One interpretation is that the nervous system begins to reach maturity near the twelfth year and the sensory systems begin to stabilize. They no longer need or benefit from such intense stimulation.

- *Students have an aversion to spinning or movement of any kind.*

  This is often due to the fact that they have poor postural stability and delayed equilibrium reactions. They do not feel as if they are able to adapt to movement. Sometimes this is a vestibular-related phenomena called "gravitational insecurity." That is, students may be able to respond to postural changes when they are on the ground, but once their feet are off the floor, their sense of position in space is impaired and they become frightened.

- *Students may begin to seizure following excessive vestibular stimulation.*

  Externally imposed vestibular stimulation is contra-indicated for students who are seizure prone.

- *Students who are not able to control the intensity of the vestibular stimulation they are receiving may become clammy to the touch, may have a slower heart rate, and may even go into shock.*

Because of the powerful, far reaching nature of the vestibular system, the visceral organs can be affected by externally imposed vestibular stimulation for up to 24 hours.

Many occupational and physical therapists are trained to use sensori-integrative therapy (S.I.). Vestibular stimulation is commonly incorporated into S.I. treatment activities. These trained therapists are fully aware of the dangers of excessive vestibular stimulation and closely monitor responses to vestibular stimulation. Although passive or externally controlled vestibular stimulation, such as spinning children in hammocks, has been a popular form of therapy, such treatment activities have largely been replaced by programming activities that require a more active role on the part of the students. Thus, students may sit in a hammock with their feet touching the floor so that they can control the speed and duration of the spinning.

Depth perception is the ability to distinguish how far one is from an object. In the past it was thought that all perceptions were the result of sensori-motor experiences. Studies with infants have revealed, however, that individuals have a built-in ability to organize certain types of stimuli. In order to perceive depth, or the distance that they are from an object, students put together information from several visual sources. These include:

(1) the accommodation/convergence mechanism of the eyes
(2) the relative distance of the eyes from each other and the resultant angles created in relation to the object
(3) brightness and shading cues
(4) the relative position of the object in relation to other objects
(5) the movement (if any) of the object and
(6) the size of the object (i. e., distant objects appear smaller to the retina) (Nelson, 1984).

When students have vision that is much better in one eye than in the other, it is likely that they will have problems perceiving depth. Conforming the visual field from one eye to the visual field of the other eye is necessary for focus and clear vision. It is also the basis for depth perception. Because the eyes are situated side-by-side, the images from the halves of each visual field are slightly offset. The brain perceives that the differences in detection of distance between the two eyes is larger for near objects than for far objects.

Teachers will notice that students with depth perception problems seem unsure when they step off curbs, move across playground equipment, or attempt balance beams or other activities that involve apparatus in the gym. To some children, stepping off a mat may seem like stepping off a three foot cliff. Stepping up onto a box one foot high may feel as though they are hopelessly suspended in space. Going down stairs may be difficult as they are unable to judge how far to step down. Getting in and out of a car may be a difficult task. When this is compounded with equilibrium problems, they may feel vulnerable and resist new activities.

PROGRAMMING FOR COMPENSATION

Teachers can help their students learn to compensate for lack of accurate visual input by exposing them to obstacle courses that provide many situations in which they must learn to adapt to objects and move their bodies in space. Typically students must go under, over, around, and through items on obstacle courses. They step down and step up. They push something along a determined distance.

Walks, field trips, and any situation in which students actively move through space should prove helpful. Experiences during table activities can also be beneficial. Students can place objects at different distances from themselves. They can place objects in shallow containers or deep containers. (Information about how proprioceptive and tactile input are related to depth perception can be found on pages 181 and 182.

Form perception is the ability to detect the shape of solid objects.

Newborn babies can distinguish lines one eighth of an inch apart and ten inches away. This means that right after birth an infant experiences a three-dimensional world. Very young babies stretch out their hands to touch solid objects. They expect to be able to manipulate visual objects. This indicates a simple unity of the visual and tactile senses. It also means that even before infants can learn about the world through motor exploration, they have the built-in ability to organize certain types of stimuli allowing them to detect shapes. As these shapes come to take on meaning they become symbols. Thus visual recognition of shapes stimulates early cognitive development.

Visual recognition of objects gives students information about the location of objects that are functional or have some special meaning. When students cannot use their vision to locate favored objects, they have less control over their own environment. They may become passive, irritable, or demanding as they experience the loss of control. They do not search or explore to the extent that is typical of students with vision. In turn, this may cause a delay in motor development, especially walking and object manipulation.

Instructional staff and other caregivers can organize their students' environment so that possessions are kept in a consistent and easily accessible location. Students should be given many and varied objects for examination, coupled with shared play activities with an adult and continuous language cues about what the object is and how it is used. Objects should be introduced in meaningful contexts; this maximizes students' ability to understand and also builds upon students' own interests.

**PROGRAMMING
FOR
COMPENSATION**

Poor body image, poor directionality, and poor laterality contribute to difficulty in perceiving relative positions in space (e.g., up, down, between, right, left, in front of, behind, over, under, etc.) of their own bodies as well as of objects.

When infants see an object in front of them, to the side of them, or to the front or back of them, they reach out for the object. Initially, this takes the form of swatting. Later they are able to grasp with two hands at midline. Visual information allows infants to "get a picture" of where things are **before** they develop cognitive concept. Eventually they can engage in one-handed, guided reaching and grasping. Processing visual information and responding to it by reaching out is cognitively less advanced then recognizing and object is there and then pursuing it. Without the visual stimulation of objects, students are not likely to attempt reaching with the same frequency. This bilateral and unilateral reaching helps to integrate the two sides of the body. The hands learn to work together and separately. Guided reaching is one way that young children learn about the relationship between their bodies and the space all around them. Movement and manipulative experiences help children to develop body image. Children who do not have many varied manipulative experiences may be delayed in establishing a hand dominance. It has also been found that a disproportionate number of individuals who experience multiple impairments are left-handed. This is true to a large extent among individuals with learning disabilities.

PROGRAMMING FOR COMPENSATION

An example of how programming can be adapted to compensate for the underlying problem would be to give students many and varied manipulative experiences with objects. Gross motor experiences have been found to be especially helpful. Simple games challenge children to use their directional skills and to differentiate between action taken by each side of the body. Obstacle courses can be fun, safe, and challenging as students move through, over, under, and around objects and across changing surfaces.

Banus B. (1971). *The developmental therapist.* Thorofare, NJ: Charles B. Slack.

Barraga, N. C. & Erin, J. N. (1992). Movement, exploration and spatial awareness. In *Visual handicaps and learning* (3rd ed.). Austin, TX: ProEd.

Erhardt, R. P. (1990). *Developmental visual dysfunction: Models of assessment and management.* Tuscon, AR: Therapy Skill Builders.

Langley, M. B. (in press). *Potential assessment of visual efficiency* (working title). Louisville, KY: American Printing House for the Blind.

Nelson, D. (1984). *Children with autism and other pervasive disorders of development and behavior.* Thorofare, NJ: Charles B. Slack.

Psychosocial Implications of Visual Impairment

Personal Factors Which Affect Psychosocial Functioning

Personal and social factors strongly influence the functioning of students who have visual impairments. When programming for these students, these factors must be taken into consideration. Restricted visual input can limit the amount of information that students receive about their environment and the people within that environment, and can limit the type and quality of experiences available to them. Without careful intervention, this isolation could result in withdrawal, self-centeredness, immaturity, mobility restrictions, a different shared frame of reference from sighted people, and over-dependence on others for information about people and events. Other personal factors could affect the students' psychological and social functioning. These could include the age of onset of the impairment, the cause of the impairment and whether it has been sudden or gradual, whether the impairment was related to a traumatic accident or event, and finally, where students are in the adjustment process.

The attitudes of others also has a significant impact on students' psychological and social adjustment. When other people reflect acceptance and support, it has a positive effect on the students' self-esteem. On the other hand, the extent to which others fear difference and perceive people with visual impairments as inferior, helpless, or to be pitied or protected can have a significant negative impact on the students' sense of self. The students' own feelings of self worth and independence are strongly tied to personal decisions about when to do things for themselves particularly when they take more time or are more difficult to do, and when to ask for help. An important way that these students can feel supported is when others communicate to them ways that they are valued, affirm their strengths, support their attempts to do things as independently as possible and provide help only when requested. This can give students a strong sense of personal control, rather than feeling that control for their lives comes from outside themselves or belong to significant others in their life.

Social Factors
Which Affect
Psychosocial
Functioning

Students who have low vision often receive mixed messages from others who are confused about whether to identify them as "blind" or "sighted". When people are unfamiliar with low vision they tend to perceive vision in black or white terms, either a person can see or cannot see. They have difficulty imagining what it is like to be able to see only a little or only under specific conditions. Consequently people may not to know whether these students are really sighted or blind and they have little frame of reference for that area in between. They may have unrealistically high or low expectations for the students. Often students who have low vision have difficulty knowing how to present themselves to others. If they portray themselves as sighted (or having low vision) people may consider them incompetent when their vision restricts their performance in a certain task. If they present themselves as legally blind they may be perceived as "faking blindness" or trying to pass as sighted when they can do a visual task which is not expected of them. Low vision students have described themselves as feeling as if they are "neither fish nor fowl", neither accepted as sighted nor accepted as blind. It takes a considerable amount of self-acceptance and patience to educate the public as to exactly what they can and cannot do. Students may want to problem solve and role play how they can communicate to others about their abilities and their needs in simple terms that they feel comfortable with. It is important that they understand that they are free to give others as much or as little information as they choose to give in any situation. They do not "owe" anyone an explanation about their disability.

Because psychological and social adjustment is so important and cannot be left to chance development, it is essential that this area of programming not be overlooked for students. *Independent Living: A Curriculum with Adaptations for Students with Visual Impairments Volume I: Social Competence* (Loumiet & Levack, 1991) addresses many of the important issues related to personal and social skills. The book is divided into goals which include interaction with family members, peers and others; developing a positive and accurate self-concept; recognizing emotions and expressing them in socially acceptable ways; using non-verbal communication; clarifying personal values; demonstrating awareness of the personal and social aspects of sexuality; demonstrating courteous behavior; demonstrating skills in problem solving, decision making and planning; developing skills for succeeding in scholastic settings; and developing a sense of personal and civic responsibility. Within each goal there is a sequence of skills which students from birth to twenty-one years of age might need. Along with the skills information is included on examples of competence, adaptations and resources for students who are visually impaired, and student books and audio-visual materials that have been written for the general population that relate to these skills.

The effect of vision loss on self esteem varies greatly from one individual to the next. It should not be assumed that all students with visual impairments have a low self esteem just as one cannot assume that all normally sighted students have a high self-esteem. Professionals who work with students who are visually impaired can use the same approach that promotes self esteem in students who are unimpaired. These include showing acceptance and appreciation for students and all that they are, providing clearly defined limits that are enforced, and allowing for individual personality differences within those limits. Mangold (1988) offers some examples of positive steps that can be taken to build self-esteem:

- **Students with visual impairments tend to believe that sighted people never spill their food, trip over furniture, or behave inappropriately.** An instructor can help a student with visual impairments realize that everyone makes mistakes by verbalizing examples of them: "I said the most embarrassing thing this morning. I don't know what came over me," or "Look at the stain on my shirt. I spilled my coffee all over myself," or "My shin is killing me from where I bumped it on the table." Students can more easily put their own mistakes into perspective if they hear about the errors others make.

- **A student with visual impairments should be given a factual explanation concerning her visual loss.** This explanation should be in age appropriate vocabulary. Sighted peers may ask questions or make negative comments about a student with visual impairments's appearance or vision loss. The negative effect of these inevitable situations can be lessened if the student with visual impairments can answer knowledgeably or respond appropriately. The most troublesome comments can be collected and used in role play to give the student practice in dealing with them.

- **Verbal and physical feedback are crucial elements of the learning process, both academically and socially.** A pat on the back and a specific description of good behavior is more effective than a smile when it is paired with pleasant voice tone to reinforce an acceptable behavior or performance. When unacceptable behavior or academic performance must be pointed out, a description of an alternative behavior or action, in specific positive terms, provides the student with useful information. The need for specific feedback applies to the student's social interactions as well. Students with visual impairments may not have learned that certain postures or mannerisms are socially unacceptable. An approach in which the student is given honest and consistent feedback that provides alternatives will be the most effective.

- **A student with visual impairments may become more independent through the use of sophisticated optical devices and electronic devices.** Those same aids and devices may contribute to a students feelings of discomfort and embarrassment. An instructor can help minimize the negative feelings about special equipment by setting up practice sessions for using the equipment in a variety of public settings. An instructor's positive feedback and encouragement can help negate the feelings of discomfort the student may have about the equipment. Instructors of young students can also introduce games into the classroom in which all the students use an optical aid of some sort to play sea captain, jeweler, detective, stamp collecting, or photographer. Classmates' discomfort or skepticism about optical devices may also be reduced if classmates are allowed to look through them. Provide interesting materials for students to inspect using the optical aid such as comic books, album covers, or colorfully detailed pictures.

- **As a student with visual impairments moves into adolescence, an unrealistic view of "normal" people as perfect socially and physically may contribute to a student's poor self image.** A student with vision loss may not realize that all teenagers suffer from self doubt, feelings of inadequacy, and a desire to "fit in" with peers. Instructors can help a student with visual impairments develop a positive self image that does not revolve around the impairment by pointing out the many variables that combine to make a personality.

Corn, A. L. (1989a). Employing critical thinking strategies within a curriculum of critical things to think about for blind and students with visual impairments. *Journal of Vision Rehabilitation, 3,* 4, 17-36.

Jose, R. T. (Ed.). (1983). Psychosocial aspects of low vision. In *Understanding low vision.* New York: American Foundation for the Blind.

Loumiet, R. & Levack, N. (1991). *Independent Living: A Curriculum with Adaptations for Students with Visual Impairments: Volume I: Social Competence.* Austin, TX: Texas School for the Blind and Visually Impaired.

Mangold, S. S. (1982). Nurturing high self-esteem in visually handicapped children. In *A teacher's guide to special education needs of blind and visually handicapped children.* New York: American Foundation for the Blind.

Mangold, S. S. (1988). Nurturing high self-esteem in adolescents with visual handicaps. *Journal of Vision Rehabilitation, 2,* 3, 5-9.

Mangold, S. S. & Mangold, P. N. (1983). The adolescent visually impaired female. *Journal of Visual Impairment and Blindness, 77,* 6, 250-255.

Read, L. F. (1989). An examination of social skills of blind kindergarten children. *Education of the Visually Handicapped, 20,* 4, 142-155.

Tuttle, D. W. (1984). *Self-esteem and adjusting with blindness: The process of responding to life's demands.* Springfield, IL: Charles Thomas.

Weisse, F. A. (1989). Self-help groups for people with vision loss. In S. L. Greenblatt (Ed.), *Providing services for people with vision loss: A multidisciplinary perspective.* Lexington, MA: Resources for Rehabilitation.

Appendices

STATE OF TEXAS
Interagency
Eye Examination Report

Patient's Name _______________________   Date of Birth _______________   Social Security No._______________

Address____   City_______________   State__________ Zip__________

Attention Eye Care Specialist
Address **each** item below.
*Your thoroughness in completing this report is essential
for this patient to receive appropriate services.*

Ocular History (e.g., previous eye diseases, injuries, or operations)

Age of onset _______________   History ____

____

Visual Acuity

If the acuity **can** be measured, complete this box using Snellen acuities or
Snellen equivalents or NLP, LP, HM, CF.

Without Glasses		With Best Correction	
Near	Distance	Near	Distance
R	R	R	R
L	L	L	L

Acuity with glare testing, if applicable: R _________   L _________

If the acuity **cannot** be measured, check
the most appropriate estimation.

☐ Legally Blind

☐ Not Legally Blind

Muscle Function   ☐ Normal   ☐ Abnormal   Describe _____________________________

Intraocular Pressure Reading   R_______________   L_______________

Visual Field Test

☐ There is no apparent visual field restriction.

☐ There **is** a field restriction.   Describe _____________________________________

☐ Yes   ☐ No   The visual field is restricted to 20 degrees or less.

Color Vision   ☐ Normal   ☐ Abnormal   **Photophobia**   ☐ Yes   ☐ No

Diagnosis (Primary cause of visual loss)

____

____

Prognosis ☐ Permanent ☐ Recurrent ☐ Improving
☐ Progressive ☐ Communicable ☐ Can Be Improved

Treatment Recommended

☐ Glasses

☐ Patches (Schedule):

R _______________________________________

L _______________________________________

☐ Medication_______________________________

☐ Refer for other medical treatment/exam:

____

☐ Low Vision Evaluation

☐ Other _______________________________________

☐ Surgery

☐ Hospitalization will be needed for approximately

_______________days.

Name of hospital_______________________________

____

Name of anesthesiologist or group:

____

Precautions or Suggestions (e.g., lighting conditions, activities to be avoided, etc.)

____

____

Scheduling Date of Next Appointment _______________________________ Time_______________

IMPORTANT **Check the most appropriate statement.**

☐ This patient appears to have no vision.

☐ This patient **has a serious visual loss** after correction.

☐ This patient **does not have** a serious visual loss after correction.

____

Print or Type Name of Licensed Ophthalmologist or Optometrist

____

Address

____

City   State   Zip

____

Signature of Licensed Ophthalmologist or Optometrist

____

Date of Examination

(_______)_______________________________

Telephone Number

RETURN COMPLETED FORM TO:

____

Name

____

Agency

____

Address

____

City   State   Zip

This form should be used when an ophthalmological/optometric examination is needed for (the): Texas Commission for the Blind (TCB) • School Districts • Special Education Programs • Regional Education Service Centers (ESCs) • Early Childhood Programs (ECH) • Early Childhood Intervention Programs (ECI) • Texas School for the Blind and Visually Impaired (TSBVI) • Eye Screening Follow-Up Examinations • Texas Department of Health (TDH) • Texas Department of Mental Health/Mental Retardation (TDMHMR).

FUNCTIONAL VISION ASSESSMENT FORM

STUDENT NAME: ______________________________ DATE OF BIRTH: ______________________________

SCHOOL: ______________________________ GRADE OR INSTRUCTIONAL LEVEL: ______________________________

EVALUATOR'S NAME: ______________________________ TITLE OR CREDENTIALS: ______________________________

DATE OF EVALUATION: ______________________________

I. MEDICAL HISTORY

General information:

____

____

Diagnosis (include acuity, field and prognosis):

____

____

Other significant impairments:

____

____

II. GENERAL OBSERVATIONS

____

____

III. OBSERVATIONS OF THE STUDENT IN FAMILIAR NEAR VISION TASKS (16 inches or less)

Instructions: Observe the student performing several familiar near vision tasks and note your observations in the appropriate columns. See page 41 for more thorough information.

Task	Describe any observed visual behaviors	Briefly describe conditions	Recommendations that might enhance visual function

During the performance of these near tasks were the following visual behaviors observed?

A. Visual Attending Behaviors (sensation)

Did the student

Yes No

1. Respond to the presence of a light, a person or an object? ☐ ☐
2. Fixate on an object or person? What? ____________________
   to the right? ☐   left? ☐   middle? ☐
3. Follow an object or person? ☐ ☐
4. Exhibit visual behaviors such as light gazing or flicking? ☐ ☐
5. Show a preferred use of the left eye? ☐ ☐
6. Show a preferred use of the right eye? ☐ ☐

B. Visual Examining Behaviors (visual cognition/perception)

Did the student

Yes No

1. React to the disappearance of an object or person? ☐ ☐
2. Search for an object or a person? ☐ ☐
3. Recognize and differentiate visual forms? ☐ ☐
4. Shift visual attention from a group of objects to a single object? ☐ ☐
5. Observe details? Of what object ____________________ ☐ ☐
6. Recognize colors? Which colors? ____________________ ☐ ☐

C. Visually Guided Motor Behaviors (visual motor)

Did the student

Yes No

1. Accurately reach for objects or people? ☐ ☐
   to the right? ☐   left? ☐   middle? ☐
2. Place objects accurately? ☐ ☐
3. Hold objects in correct position after looking at how they should be positioned? What kind of objects? ____________________ ☐ ☐

   ____
4. Turn or tilt her head for eccentric viewing? ☐ ☐
   Describe how the head was tilted. ____________________

   ____

IV. OBSERVATIONS OF STUDENTS IN FAMILIAR INTERMEDIATE (16" to 3') AND DISTANCE (3' or More) VISION TASKS

Instructions: *Observe the student performing several familiar intermediate vision tasks and several familiar distance tasks and note observations in the appropriate columns. See page 42 in the resource guide for more thorough information.*

Task	Describe any observed visual behaviors	Briefly describe conditions including distance between student and task	Recommendations that might enhance visual functioning

During the performance of these intermediate and distance tasks were the following visual behaviors observed?

A. Visual Attending Behaviors (sensation)

Did the student   Yes   No

1. Fixate on an object or person? ☐ ☐
   What? _____________ At what distances? _________

2. Search for an object or a person? ☐ ☐
   What? _____________ At what distances? _________

3. Follow an object or person? ☐ ☐
   What? _____________ At what distances? _________

4. React to an object or person in the periphery? ☐ ☐
   Left? ☐   Right? ☐   Above? ☐   Below? ☐

B. Visual Examining Behaviors (visual cognition/perception)

Did the student   Yes   No

1. React to the disappearance of an object or person? ☐ ☐
   At what distances? _________

2. Shift gaze from one object or person to another? ☐ ☐
   Describe the size of the objects and the distances. _____________

   ____

3. Identify objects? ☐ ☐
   Describe the size of the object and the distance. _____________

   ____

C. Visually Guided Motor Behaviors (visual motor)

Did the student   Yes   No

1. Move successfully within a familiar environment? ☐ ☐
   What environment? _____________________________

2. Imitate movements?   At what distance? _________ ☐ ☐

   Describe: ______________________________________

3. Notice drop offs, slopes, and step-ups? ☐ ☐

   Describe: ______________________________________

4. Move successfully in an unfamiliar environment? ☐ ☐

5. Was there any area in the student's visual field that seemed to be a problem, such as bumping into objects while travelling? ☐ ☐

   Describe the area: ______________________________

V. ACADEMIC CONSIDERATIONS

This section should be completed only if the student is doing some academic seatwork.

1. Reading print	Observation	Recommendations
a. Low vision devices used		
b. Smallest readable size of print	☐ 9 pt. ☐ 10 pt. ☐ 12 pt. ☐ 14 pt. ☐ 16 pt. ☐ 18 pt. ☐ 20 pt. ☐ 24 pt. ☐ _____	
c. Preferred size of print Reading speed ____________	☐ 9 pt. ☐ 10 pt. ☐ 12 pt. ☐ 14 pt. ☐ 16 pt. ☐ 18 pt. ☐ 20 pt. ☐ 24 pt. ☐ _____	
d. Use of contrast (e.g., dittos, copies, colored paper)		
e. Preferred format of written material (e.g., white space, illustrations)		
f. Means of maintaining one's place when reading		

2. *Writing or Drawing*	Observation	Recommendations
a. Type of paper and preferred writing implement (e.g., green lined paper, black felt pen)		
b. Low vision devices used		
c. Writing aids and other assistance (e.g., signature guide)		
d. Writing activities that require extra time		

3. Describe the student''s ability to use regular textbooks and workbooks.

____

____

____

4. Describe the student''s ability to read and copy from the blackboard and any adaptations that are needed.

____

____

____

5. Describe the student's ability to view projected images in the classroom and any adaptations that are needed.

6. Describe the student's ability to observe classroom demonstrations and any adaptations that are needed.

7. Describe the student's ability to scan rooms (e.g., auditorium, cafeteria, classroom) and any adaptations that are needed.

8. Describe the student's ability to locate objects in the classroom and any adaptations that are needed.

9. Describe the student's ability to organize personal belongings, books, school supplies, etc.

VI. ENVIRONMENTAL CONDITIONS

	Yes	No	Observations

1. Does the student adjust to sudden changes from light to dark? ☐ Yes ☐ No — If so, how much time is needed for the adjustment?

2. Does the student have more difficulty in bright conditions? ☐ Yes ☐ No

   in darkened conditions? ☐ Yes ☐ No

3. What type of illumination is most helpful? ☐ Yes ☐ No

4. Does the student discriminate figure ground in visually cluttered environments? ☐ Yes ☐ No

5. Are there any particular problems with indoor travel and functioning? ☐ Yes ☐ No

6. Are there any particular problems with outdoor travel and functioning? ☐ Yes ☐ No

7. Are there any problems with night vision or a darkened environment? ☐ Yes ☐ No

8. Does the student have difficulty with fluctuating visual abilities? ☐ Yes ☐ No — If so, what conditions contribute to this?

9. Are there any environmental situations where the student seems to perform with less ability? ☐ Yes ☐ No

VII. INFORMAL VISUAL ACUITY TESTING

1. What assessment item(s) were used)?

2. Did the student use   prescription lenses?   Yes ☐ ____________________ No ☐

   (Describe.)   low vision device(s)?   Yes ☐ ____________________ No ☐

      non-optical device(s)?   Yes ☐ ____________________ No ☐

3. Describe the lighting conditions

4. Near vision acuity results: ____________________   Distance vision acuity results: ____________________

5. Additional comments:

VIII. Recommendations

A. In your opinion does the student meet the eligibility criteria as visually handicapped?   Yes ☐   No ☐

B. What instructional services would you recommend related to the student's visual handicap?

Type of instruction	Purpose	By whom	Recommended frequency and duration

C. Are there additional evaluations that you would recommend (e. g., clinical low vision, oriemtation and mobility)?

Type of evaluation	By whom	Reason for recommendation

D. Do you recommend that the student be registered to receive any of the following services? (Check all that apply.)

☐ Consultative and technical assistance from regional education service center

☐ Texas Commission for the Blind Children's services, educational aids

☐ Textbooks in ☐ Braille ☐ Large Print ☐ Audio

☐ Texas State Library Supplemental reading materials, cassette player/recorder

☐ Other:_______________________

215

E. As a result of this functional assessment, please give recommendations for instructional strategies and environmental adaptations. (Check all that apply.)

The student's primary mode of learning is ☐ visual, ☐ auditory, ☐ tactual.

☐ Sighted guide or assistance is needed when travelling.

Specify what kind of assistance __________

☐ Special considerations for classroom organization are needed.

Specify__________

☐ Special considerations for changes in routine or disaster drills are needed.

Specify__________

☐ Time modifications are needed.

Specify__________

☐ Positioning considerations for student and materials are needed.

Specify__________

☐ Low vision devices should be clinically evaluated.

Specify__________

☐ Physical education modifications are needed.

Specify__________

☐ Other environmental modifications are needed.

Specify__________

☐ Other instructional materials or equipment are needed.

Specify__________

FUNCTIONAL VISION ASSESSMENT FORM

STUDENT NAME: *P. C.*

DATE OF BIRTH: *10-17-81*

SCHOOL: *SISD*

GRADE OR INSTRUCTIONAL LEVEL: *4*

EVALUATOR'S NAME: *M. E.*

TITLE OR CREDENTIALS: *VH Teacher*

DATE OF EVALUATION: *11/91*

I. MEDICAL HISTORY

General information:

Normal development until head trauma at age one. Damage to brain resulted in vision loss.

Diagnosis (include acuity, field and prognosis):

Cortical visual impairment

Other significant impairments:

Motor planning impairment / Difficulty producing speech on demand (anomia) / Poor coordination, balance / Some specific learning disabilities (auditory processing)

II. GENERAL OBSERVATIONS

Limited interaction with peers, poor self concept, very dependent on particular staff person for direction, very odd eating habits, reading above instructional level, does not dress self, tries very hard

III. OBSERVATIONS OF THE STUDENT IN FAMILIAR NEAR VISION TASKS (16 inches or less) SAMPLE

Instructions: Observe the student performing several familiar near vision tasks and note your observations in the appropriate columns. See page 41 for more thorough information.

Task	Describe any observed visual behaviors	Briefly describe conditions	Recommendations that might enhance visual function
Map reading	Moves materials around as	Sat at table.	Use reading stand so that
Picture interpretation	though trying to find	Normal fluorescent	head does not block light.
Reading	optimum distance, angle.	lighting	Refer for clinical low vision
Writing	Settles on 2"-4" viewing--	No low vision devices	evaluation.
Art (creating designs	left eye primarily.		Magnification does not
with pegs, design	Field appears to be very		appear to be helpful.
copy)	restricted. Reads large		Are we sure refraction is
	print one letter at a time		O.K.?
	with head movement		
	from letter to letter.		
	Figure-ground problems		
	with photos. Was able		
	to identify major subjects.		
	Was not able to		
	interpret melieu.		

During the performance of these near tasks were the following visual behaviors observed?

A. Visual Attending Behaviors
(sensation)

Did the student

1. Respond to the presence of a light, a person or an object?   Yes ☑ No ☐

2. Fixate on an object or person? What? ______________   Yes ☑ No ☐
   to the right? ☑   left? ☑   middle? ☑

3. Follow an object or person?   Yes ☑ No ☐

4. Exhibit visual behaviors such as light gazing or flicking?   Yes ☐ No ☑

5. Show a preferred use of the left eye?   Yes ☑ No ☐

6. Show a preferred use of the right eye?   Yes ☐ No ☑

B. Visual Examining Behaviors
(visual cognition/perception)

Did the student

1. React to the disappearance of an object or person?   Yes ☑ No ☐

2. Search for an object or a person?   Yes ☑ No ☐

3. Recognize and differentiate visual forms?   Yes ☑ No ☐

4. Shift visual attention from a group of objects to a single object?   Yes ☑ No ☐

5. Observe details? Of what object _Letters, #s, pictures, toys_   Yes ☑ No ☐

6. Recognize colors? Which colors? _all_   Yes ☑ No ☐

C. Visually Guided Motor Behaviors
(visual motor)

Did the student

1. Accurately reach for objects or people? _Hesitantly, some_   Yes ☑ No ☐
   to the right? ☐   left? ☐   middle? ☐ _overreaching_

2. Place objects accurately?   Yes ☑ No ☐

3. Hold objects in correct position after looking at how they should   Yes ☑ No ☐
   be positioned? What kind of objects?
   Pen, pegs, books, maps

4. Turn or tilt her head for eccentric viewing?   Yes ☑ No ☐
   Describe how the head was tilted. _Placed left eye within 1-4"_
   of object. Moved object and head up & down

IV. OBSERVATIONS OF STUDENTS IN FAMILIAR INTERMEDIATE (16" to 3') AND DISTANCE (3' or More) VISION TASKS

Instructions: Observe the student performing several familiar intermediate vision tasks and several familiar distance tasks and note observations in the appropriate columns. See page 42 in the resource guide for more thorough information.

Task	Describe any observed visual behaviors	Briefly describe conditions including distance between student and task	Recommendations that might enhance visual functioning
Loading braille writer	Followed 1" masking tape	Normal fluorescent light	Needs stimulus reduction in
Hanging coat	path - curved, turns,	No low vision devices	all environments.
Putting away work	without bending over.	Distances, etc., noted in	Needs maximum contrast.
materials	Tan tape on orange	previous column.	Movement of object helps
Playing catch	carpet. Viewing distance		perception.
Driving cars on tape	4' - 6 '. Read cards		Clinical low vision evaluation
Following tape path	at 10/100 o. u. Able to		Telescope?
Lighthouse cards	track white 1/4" ball		
	rolled to him on orange		
	carpet from 6' away when		
	rolled to both right and		
	left sides.		
	Much head movement and		
	searching when asked to		
	find stationary ball.		
	Figure-ground problem		
	with coat hanging.		

During the performance of these intermediate and distance tasks were the following visual behaviors observed?

A. Visual Attending Behaviors (sensation)

Did the student   Yes No
1. Fixate on an object or person? ☑ ☐
   What? _Everything_   At what distances?_Person 20'_
   1" stationary ball 6'
2. Search for an object or a person? ☑ ☐
   What? _Everything_   At what distances?_see above_
3. Follow an object or person? ☑ ☐
   What? _Ball, track, person_   At what distances?_See IV_
4. React to an object or person in the periphery? ☑ ☐
   Left? ☑   Right? ☐   Above? ☐   Below? ☑

B. Visual Examining Behaviors (visual cognition/perception)

Did the student   Yes No
1. React to the disappearance of an object or person? ☑ ☐
   At what distances?_See #1_
2. Shift gaze from one object or person to another? ☑ ☐
   Describe the size of the objects and the distances. _See #1_
3. Identify objects? ☑ ☐
   Describe the size of the object and the distance. _2" toy car, 1" toy fork at 4"_

C. Visually Guided Motor Behaviors (visual motor)

Did the student   Yes No
1. Move successfully within a familiar environment? ☑ ☐
   What environment?_whole school_
2. Imitate movements?   At what distance?_5'_ ☑ ☐
   Describe:_Hand movements, sitting, standing_
3. Notice drop offs, slopes, and step-ups? ☑ ☐
   Describe:_Changes in color perceived as drop off_
4. Move successfully in an unfamiliar environment? _Avoided obstacles - unable to orient._ ☐ ☑
5. Was there any area in the student's visual field that seemed to be a problem, such as bumping into objects while travelling? ☐ ☑
   Describe the area:

V. ACADEMIC CONSIDERATIONS

This section should be completed only if the student is doing some academic seatwork.

SAMPLE

1. Reading print	Observation	Recommendations
a. Low vision devices used	CCTV - did not help. Field too large.	
b. Smallest readable size of print	☐ 9 pt. ☐ 10 pt. ☑ 12 pt.　☐ 14 pt. ☐ 16 pt. ☐ 18 pt.　☐ 20 pt. ☐ 24 pt. ☐ ____	
c. Preferred size of print Reading speed	☐ 9 pt. ☐ 10 pt. ☐ 12 pt.　☐ 14 pt. ☐ 16 pt. ☑ 18 pt.　☐ 20 pt. ☐ 24 pt. ☐ ____	
d. Use of contrast (e.g., dittos, copies, colored paper)	Used dittos if size large enough. Was able to follow lines on print map, recognize regions by color.	
e. Preferred format of written material (e.g., white space, illustrations)	Needs maximum spacing; even between letters of a word. Likes color illustrations.	
f. Means of maintaining one's place when reading	Visually scans page for initial orientation. Reads letter by letter so slowly, content gets lost.	Braille: Reading, lang.arts, soc.st., science. Print: Math. Print & braille: Spelling. Pair with print partner for access to illustrations. Give all worksheets in braille and print.

2. *Writing or Drawing*	Observation	Recommendations
a. Type of paper and preferred writing implement (e.g., green lined paper, black felt pen)	*Unlined paper, pencil preferred, but not optimum. Letters are unrecognizable. Numbers are O.K. Likes to draw.*	*Should continue to draw. Drawings are meaningful to him.*
b. Low vision devices used		
c. Writing aids and other assistance (e.g., signature guide)		*Try green lines paper, Erasermate pen*
d. Writing activities that require extra time	*All*	*Continue to do math in pen and paper mode. Perhaps spelling & multiple choice tests as well.*

3. **Describe the student''s ability to use regular textbooks and workbooks.**

   Needs 12 point, good spacing. Uses print mainly for illustrations. Print worksheets sometimes helpful, if not too busy.

4. **Describe the student''s ability to read and copy from the blackboard and any adaptations that are needed.**

   Not now. Maybe with telescope later.

5. **Describe the student's ability to view projected images in the classroom and any adaptations that are needed.**

Not able to do this.

6. **Describe the student's ability to observe classroom demonstrations and any adaptations that are needed.**

Needs stimulus reduction. Can see science experiment at 5" if it is desk top size.

7. **Describe the student's ability to scan rooms (e.g., auditorium, cafeteria, classroom) and any adaptations that are needed.**

Moves head to search for specific landmarks.

8. **Describe the student's ability to locate objects in the classroom and any adaptations that are needed.**

Moves to general area where object is kept. Sometimes unable to find object in spite of searching if areas is cluttered.

9. **Describe the student's ability to organize personal belongings, books, school supplies, etc.**

Does not have enough room to store all materials.

VI. ENVIRONMENTAL CONDITIONS

#	Question	Yes	No	Observations
1.	Does the student adjust to sudden changes from light to dark?		✓	If no, how much time is needed for adjustment?
2.	Does the student have more difficulty in bright conditions?		✓	
	in darkened conditions?	✓		*Can't see in dim light.*
3.	What type of illumination is most helpful?			*Normal outdoor. Normal fluorescent indoor.*
4.	Does the student discriminate figure ground in visually cluttered environments?		✓	
5.	Are there any particular problems with indoor travel and functioning?	✓		*Reduced field. Much searching, confusion. Needs extra time. Appears insecure.*
6.	Are there any particular problems with outdoor travel and functioning?	✓		*Same. Partly cloudy days, shadows produce more confusion.*
7.	Are there any problems with night vision or a darkened environment?	✓		*Very non-functional in darkened room. Not observed at night.*
8.	Does the student have difficulty with fluctuating visual abilities?	✓		If so, what conditions contribute to this? *Some seems organic. Other factors previously noted.*
9.	Are there any environmental situations where the student seems to perform with less ability?	✓		*Clutter, dark, shadows.*

VII. INFORMAL VISUAL ACUITY TESTING

1. What assessment item(s) were used)?

   Lighthouse cards.

2. Did the student use   prescription lenses?   Yes ☐   No ☑

   (Describe.)   low vision device(s)?   Yes ☐   No ☑

      non-optical device(s)? Yes ☐   No ☑

3. Describe the lighting conditions

   Normal fluorescent.

4. Near vision acuity results: *12 pt. at 2" - 4"*   Distance vision acuity results: *10/100 o.u.*

5. Additional comments:

   Vision fluctuates. Performance noted is average.

VIII. Recommendations

A. In your opinion does the student meet the eligibility criteria as visually handicapped?   Yes ☑   No

B. What instructional services would you recommend related to the student's visual handicap?

Type of instruction	Purpose	By whom	Recommended frequency and duration
Reading, math, language arts,	braille, abacus, Braille 'N	VH itinerant teacher	1 hr. daily direct,
social studies, science	Speak, visual adaptations		1 hr. daily adaptations
	of maps, worksheets	Regular ed. teacher	

C. Are there additional evaluations that you would recommend (e. g., clinical low vision, orientation and mobility)?

Type of evaluation	By whom	Reason for recommendation
Clinical low vision evaluation	ophthalmologist/optometrist	use of telescope?
Motor	OT/PT	motor-planning problems
Psychological	Psychol./Ed. Diagnostician	auditory processing
Speech/Language	Speech Pathologist	anomia

D. Do you recommend that the student be registered to receive any of the following services? (Check all that apply.)

☑ Consultative and technical assistance from regional education service center

☑ Texas Commission for the Blind
Children's services, educational aids

☑ Textbooks in ☑ Braille
☑ Large Print
☐ Audio

☑ Texas State Library
Supplemental reading materials, cassette player/recorder

☐ Other:_______________

E. As a result of this functional assessment, please give recommendations for instructional strategies and environmental adaptations. (Check all that apply.)

The student's primary mode of learning is ☑ visual, ☐ auditory, ☑ tactual.

☑ Sighted guide or assistance is needed when travelling.

Specify what kind of assistance _Verbal explanation of misperceived drop-offs in unfamiliar environments. Verbal orientation prompts in unfamiliar environments._

☑ Special considerations for classroom organization are needed.

Specify _Access to special tools and materials. More storage for books._

☑ Special considerations for changes in routine or disaster drills are needed.

Specify _May not be aware of blockage or know how to re-orient to different route._

☑ Time modifications are needed.

Specify _Field restriction paired with size enhancement means print materials are consumed very slowly._

☑ Positioning considerations for student and materials are needed.

Specify _Reading stand for near work. Needs to be about 5" from stimulus at distance._

☑ Low vision devices should be clinically evaluated.

Specify _Maybe telescope?_

☑ Physical education modifications are needed.

Specify _More related to motor problems than vision._

☑ Other environmental modifications are needed.

Specify _Stimulus reduction, good light, high contrast (color enhancement)._

☐ Other instructional materials or equipment are needed.

Specify ____

Distance Test Chart for the Partially Sighted Person
>Black numbers on white heavy plastic sheets
>*Designs for Vision*
>For students who cannot respond to the Snellen Chart at 20'.
>Also used to provide more than one symbol at each level of
>the lower acuities. In addition it is used to provide acuities
>between those found on standard Snellen charts, e. g.,
>acuities between 20/100 and 20/200

Teller Acuity Cards
>*Vistech*
>For infants and non-verbal, multiply handicapped students
>functioning at 3-18 months level; special training required

Standard 20-Foot Eye Charts
>Black Snellen optotype letters from 20/200 to 20/10. Black on
>white plastic.
>*The Lighthouse Low Vision Products*

HOTV Children's Distance Vision Eye Test Kit
>White plastic cards and response panels with optotype letters
>that can be illuminated from front or back
>*Good-Lite*

20-Foot Distance Symbol Eye Chart for Children
>House, apple, umbrella on white chart or individual cards
>black on white plastic.
>*The Lighthouse Low Vision Products*
>For non-readers who can match, imitate, and point

Pediatric Low Vision Test Chart
>Black drawings of objects on white heavy plastic (more
>detailed than Snellen chart)
>*Designs for Vision*

STYCAR Vision Tests: Flip Cards, Letter Chart, "Panda" Test
>*Institute of Psychological Research*
>For non-readers who can match, imitate, and point; can be
>used as young as 6 mos., but does not give exact acuity

**INSTRUMENTS TO
MEASURE
CENTRAL ACUITY
THAT IS LESS
THAN 20'**

STYCAR Vision Tests: Rolling Balls, Toys
　　Institute of Psychological Research
　　For children who cannot interpret 2-D symbols

INSTRUMENTS TO MEASURE CENTRAL ACUITY AT NEARPOINT (i. e., READING DISTANCE)

Lighthouse Near Visual Acuity Test
　　Designed with Sloan letters for testing subnormal vision at
　　　　40cm/16 in. Black letters from distant equivalents 5/200 -
　　　　20/25 (or 40 - 1 diopters) on white heavy plastic.
　　The Lighthouse Low Vision Products
　　For students who can identify letters

Sloan Continuous-Text for Adults and Children
　　Continuous text cards with courier type on white plastic
　　　　flashcards (8x10) for 1 m to 20 m.
　　The Lighthouse Low Vision Products
　　For students who can read at least at 2nd grade level

Jaeger Test Card
　　Bernell
　　For school-age children who can identify symbols (pictures,
　　　　letters, words)

Tumbling E/Tumbling Hands Card
　　Bernell
　　For non-readers who can match, imitate, and point

Wells Standard Test Types Card
　　Bernell

Assortment of colored pieces of paper in pairs or more
    School or Classroom Supply
    For all ages

Holmgren Wool Test
    For adults

Knowlton & Woo Functional Color Assessment
    For school age students

Ishihara Plates
    Bernell

Amsler Chart Manual
    Seven charts to evaluate color and line distortions.
    The Lighthouse Low Vision Products

STYCAR Balls (white balls on black wands)
    Institute of Psychological Research

Stereoscopic Vision Screening
    Titmus

Stereo Fly Test
    Bernell

Stereo Reindeer Test
    Bernell

Motor-Free Visual Perception Test (MVPT)
    Pro•Ed

Random Dot E Test
    Bernell

Diagnostic Assessment Procedure (DAP)
    American Printing House for the Blind
    Best with young children with a functional age of 3 years or
        older, hardest items are appropriate for 6-7 years. Lower
        elementary interest level

INSTRUMENTS TO MEASURE COLOR PERCEPTION

INSTRUMENTS TO MEASURE FIELD OF VISION

INSTRUMENTS TO MEASURE STEREOPSIS

INSTRUMENTS TO MEASURE VISUAL EFFICIENCY & PERCEPTION

INSTRUMENTS TO MEASURE CONTRAST

Vision Contrast Test System
   Grey cricles in varying shades with left, right, and up lines.
   VisTech

Optokinetic drum
   House of Vision Instrument Co.

For addresses and phone numbers please consult the *Directory of Services for Blind and Visually Impaired Persons in the United States* (1988) or the *International Low Vision Directory* (Yeadon, 1988).

accommodation	the adjustment of the eye for seeing at different distances which is achieved through changing the shape of the lens
acuity	measurement of the sharpness of vision as it relates to the ability to discriminate detail
adaptation	modification or adjustment to compensate for a disability
Admission, Review and Dismissal Committee meeting (ARD) *adventitious*	the annual meeting of the student's parents and educational team which develops, reviews, and revises the Individual Education Plan (IEP), must be held for each student who has been identified as having a handicapping condition occurring after birth
adventitious visual impairment	a visual impairment that was acquired after visual memory was established and the person has some visual concepts and skills
afocal	unable to be focused
amniocentesis	a procedure in which amniotic fluid is drawn from the womb and tested to determine if the fetus has chromosomal abnormalities
anoxia	a lack of oxygen
anterior	situated near or toward the head, front
aphakia	the absence of the lens of the eye which results from surgery or is a congenital impairment
ASCII code	acronym for *American Standard Code for Information Interchange;* pronounced "ASK-ee" in which the numbers from 0 to 127 stand for text and control characters.
assessment	the procedure used to determine the student's present levels of functioning
ataxia	an inability to coordinate voluntary muscular movements that is symptomatic of some nervous disorders, unsteadiness of gait

athetosis	a condition of the nerves supplying the muscles which causes slow, twisting, continuous and involuntary movements
autosomal	referring to or characteristic of a non-sex-determining chromosome
bilateral	having or affecting two sides
binocular vision	coordinated use of both eyes to focus on the same object and see a single three dimensional object
blue sclera	an abnormality in which the sclera is thin and has a blue appearance because the underlying pigmented choroid shows through the thin sclera
braille	a system of reading using raised dots which is used by some people who cannot see well enough to read print
CAT scan	computer assisted tomography, use of X-rays to look for lesions in the eye's orbit or brain
cataract	a condition in which the lens of the eye becomes opaque, resulting in loss of acuity
closed circuit television (CCTV)	a device that allows an individual to see printed material on a television screen, illuminated and magnified to preferred degree
color deficiency	partial or complete inability to discriminate colors
congenital	present at birth
contact lenses	lenses made to fit directly on the cornea
contractures	a permanent shortening of a muscle or tendon which produces deformity or distortion
contrast	the apparent difference between foreground and background in terms of color or shading which enables items to be seen better
cortical	related to the cerebral cortex of the brain

critical moment	the time during the performance of a task during which continuous visual contact on the materials of the task is necessary
cryotherapy	treatment by cold usually involving the freezing of the tissue concerned
depth perception	the perception of three-dimensionality and relative distance of objects from the viewer
device	lens or telescope designed to help students who have low vision to help them see objects at a distance, read small print, or do close work
diffused light	light that is spread out and covers a large area
diopters	units of measurement used to determine lens power and refraction
direct light	light that is not shielded; often causes glare
distance vision	the ability to see objects clearly from far away
dominant	a gene whose effect on the visible characteristics of an individual completely obscures the effect of other gene in the pair
drop-off	the point at which a surface level becomes lower at a sharp angle
dwarfism	short stature associated with a number of syndromes
eccentric viewing	an adaptive process which involves using the operative part of the retina when obstructions occur, such as turning the head to look out of the side of the eye
enucleation	surgical removal of the eyeball
evaluation	a procedure to determine levels of functioning
extension	a movement between two connecting bones that increases the angle between them (e. g., straightening an arm)
extensor	one of the muscles of the forearm or of the calf of the leg

extraocular	outside of the eye
fascia	a sheet of connective tissue covering or binding body structures together
fixate	to direct a gaze and hold an object steadily in view
flexion	a movement between two connecting bones that decreases the angle between them (e. g., bringing an arm to the chest)
flexor	a muscle of the forearm
flicking	a self-stimulatory behavior in which the hand, fingers, or an object is rapidly waved back and forth in front of the eye, may take place to the exclusion of other more meaningful visual activities
functional vision	see *low vision*
functional vision assessment	a determination of how an individual uses vision in daily activities and/or under specific conditions
gaze	to fix the eyes in a steady and intent look
gene	a unit of heredity which occupies a specific position in a chromosome and either alone or in combination produces a single characteristic
glare	light that causes the eye discomfort
hypertonic	exhibiting excessive tone or tension
hypoplasia	an incomplete or underdeveloped organ or tissue
hypotonic	having deficient tone or tension
IEP	Individual Education Plan, a written plan of instruction for a student who receives special education services; must include present levels of the student's educational performance, annual goals, short-term objectives, and specific services that the student will need

illumination	the amount and type of light that falls on a surface
intra-ocular	inside the eye
learning media	the materials or methods that students use in conjunction with their sensory channels to get information
legal blindness	acuity of 20/200 or less in the better eye with best possible correction or a field of 20° or less diameter in the better eye
lesions	a wound, injury or other damage to body tissue
light gazing	a self- stimulatory behavior in which visual attention is directed at a light source to the exclusion of other visual stimuli; individuals may engage in "flicking" while light gazing to increase sensory stimulation
light perception	the ability to distinguish light from dark
light projection	the ability to determine where light is coming from
literary medium	a subset or component of learning media which is based on the sensory channel the student will use for reading and writing (e. g., print or braille)
loupes	telescopes or other lenses mounted on spectacles to provide additional magnification for close work
low vision	having a significant visual impairment but also having some usable vision; moderate low vision is acuity of 20/70 to 20/160 in the better eye with the best possible correction; severe vision loss is 20/200 to 20/400 or a visual field of 20° or less
low vision device	see *device*

low vision clinic	a clinic in which vision is assessed, low vision aids and devices are prescribed, and instructions are given on how to use them
low vision programming	an overall plan of instruction for a student with low vision
mannerism	see *stereotypical behavior*
microcephaly	a condition in which the head and the brain are unusually small
mobility	the ability to navigate from one position in the environment to another
monocular	a hand-held telescope prescribed for use with one eye
multi-sensory approach	educational programming in which all sensory capacities are considered and used in combination to enhance learning
near point of	the point closest to the bridge of the nose where
convergence	convergence and binocular singular vision can no longer be maintained as the object approaches
near vision	the ability to see objects clearly at normal reading distance
neurological	related to the nervous system
neuromuscular	related to the nerves that affect the muscles
null point	distance from the position of the eyes where nystagmus is dampened or minimal
ophthalmologist	a medical doctor who specializes in the diagnosis and treatment of eye diseases and defects and prescribes glasses, contact lenses, prism lenses and/or exercises, and performs surgery
optician	a technician who grinds lenses and prepares eyeglasses, and fits contact lenses from prescriptions from ophthalmologists and optometrists

optometrist	a non-medical practitioner who measures refractive errors and eye muscle imbalances and prescribes glasses, contact lenses, prism lenses, and/or exercises
orientation	the process of using the senses to establish position in space and relationship to other objects in the environment
orientation & mobility	a field of instruction which teaches systematic techniques of travel and orientation to people who are blind or visually impaired
partial participation	the technique of allowing a student with limited ability to participate in an activity as much as possible so that the student can gain experience and confidence
perception	the ability to understand sensory information
peripheral vision	the perception of objects or motion from the parts of the retina that are beyond the macula
photophobia	extreme sensitivity to light or discomfort from light
posterior	the part that is to the back or behind
prism	a transparent, solid piece of optical material, often wedge shaped that bends rays of light toward its base without converging or diverging parallel rays
proprioception	a feeling which is linked to cues from within the body that helps one to know the position of the body parts and motions of the muscles and joints
ptosis	a paralytic drooping of the upper eyelid
radiography	the use of radiation (e. g., X-rays) to make images on photographic film
range of motion	the natural direction that an arm or leg would move

reading stand	a support for a book that allows for adjustment of the book to a comfortable position for the reader
recessive	a gene whose effect on the visible characteristics is largely or entirely obscured by the effect of the other gene in the pair
reflex	the unwilling working or movement of an organ or part of a body in response to a specific action, usually occurs without thinking
reticular activating system (RAS)	a working system in the brain needed for the level of consciousness from sleep to full attention
rheostat control	a light switch that allows for infinitely variable adjustments of brightness
scanning	a systematic and coordinated use of the head and eyes to search for objects in the environment
scotoma	a blind or partially blind area in the visual field
spasticity	paralysis with tonic spasm of the affected muscles with increased tendon reflexes
stereopsis	the perception of objects in space and their relative position to one another
stereotypical behavior	an activity that a student performs repeatedly because it is satisfying or soothing (e.g., rocking, eye poking, hand waving or ringing, head rocking, object flicking)
subcortical	related to, involving, or being nerve centers below the cerebral cortex
subluxation	a condition of the muscles not holding the bones in position in the shoulder girdle and spine
syndrome	a group of symptoms that occur together that may affect the whole body or any of its parts

telemicroscope   an optical aid used for near vision tasks

telescope   an optical aid used for visual tasks at a distance

tracking   a systematic use of the eyes to follow an object or print

trailing   a method of gathering information and travelling that uses either ones hand or a cane

transdisciplinary service delivery model   specialists from a variety of fields (e.g., occupational therapy, physical therapy, sensory impairments , speech and language) work together with the parents and student to provide a meaningful and functional program for the student

trisomy   the existence of three chromosomes of one variety rather than the normal pair of chromosomes

tunnel vision   a condition in which the visual field is contracted to such an extent that only a small area of central visual acuity is left, giving the affected individual the impression of looking through a tunnel

typoscope   a piece of black cardboard with a slit to block out all but the line of print that can be viewed through the slit and increasing contrast for the print that is exposed

visual acuity   the ability to see clearly and discriminate detail

visual attending   the act of maintaining visual contact over a period of time

visual clutter   objects or patterns in the field of vision which cause visual conflict or confusion

visual coding   the strategic addition of visual cues that will significantly facilitate task performance

visual conspicuity   the capacity of a visual stimulus to attract attention

visual cue control	the regulation of the visual stimuli presented
visual examining	visual cognitive component, using the eyes to inspect and gain meaningful information about objects
visual field	the entire area that can be seen without shifting the eyes or moving the head
visual functioning	how individuals use their ability to see and interpret what is seen
visually guided motor behaviors	visual motor), movements that result from, or are guided by, visual input
visual impairment	identified organic differences in the visual system which are so severe that even after medical and conventional optical intervention, the student is unable to receive an appropriate education within the regular educational setting without special education services
visually impaired	used in this resource guide to refer to individuals who are blind and individuals who have low vision
X-linked	refers to genes on the X chromosome

Aitken, S. & Buultjens, M. (1991). Visual assessments of children with multiple impairments: A survey of ophthalmologists. *Journal of Visual Impairment and Blindness, 85,* 4, 170-173.

Angelucci, A., DeCaluwe, S., Kukla, D., Peck, P., & Strand, C. (n. d.) *Early vision stimulation.* Unpublished paper.

Arensman, D. (1975). The role of the teacher for visually handicapped in vision assessment. *Education of the Visually Handicapped, 7,* I, 5-7.

Bailey, I, L. (1978). Visual field measurement in low vision. *Optometric Monthly, 7,* 84-88.

Bailey, I. L. & Hall, A. (1990). *Visual impairment: An overview.* New York: American Foundation for the Blind.

Baldasare, J., Watson, G. R., Whittaker, S. G., & Miller-Shafer, I. H. (1986). The development and evaluation of a reading test for low vision individuals with macular loss. *Journal of Visual Impairment and Blindness, 80,* 6, 785-789.

Banus, B. (1971). *The developmental therapist.* Thorofare, NJ: Charles B. Slack.

Barraga, N. C. (n. d.). *Activities to promote visual development in low vision children.* Unpublished paper.

Barraga, N. C. (n. d.). *A programmatic approach to visual learning and utilization of low vision.* Unpublished paper.

Barraga, N. C. (n. d.). *Sequence of visual development.* Unpublished paper.

Barraga, N. C. (1964). *Increased visual behavior in low vision children.* New York: American Foundation for the Blind.

Barraga, N. C. (1969). *Learning efficiency in low vision.* Unpublished paper.

Barraga, N. C. (1970). *Teacher's guide for development of visual learning abilities and utilization of low vision.* Louisville, KY: American Printing House for the Blind.

Barraga, N. C. (1983). *Visual handicaps and learning* (rev. ed.). Austin, TX: Exceptional Resources.

Barraga, N. C. & Collins, M., E. (1979). Development of efficiency in visual functioning: Rationale for comprehensive programming. *Journal of Visual Impairment and Blindness, 73,* 4, 121-126.

Barraga, N. C., Collins, M. E., & Hollis, J. (1977). Development of efficiency in visual functioning: A literature analysis. *Journal of Visual Impairment and Blindness, 74,* 3, 93-96.

Barraga, N. C. & Erin, J. N. (1992). *Visual handicaps and learning* (3rd ed.). Austin, TX: Pro•Ed.

Barraga, N. C. & Morris, J. E. (1980). *Program to develop efficiency in visual functioning: Source book on low vision.* Louisville, KY: American Printing House for the Blind.

Basso, L. V., (1978). The condition known as diabetes mellitus. *Journal of Visual Impairment and Blindness, 72,* 9, 338-342.

Beatty, L. A. (1991). The effects of visual impairment on adolescents' self-concept. *Journal of Visual Impairment and Blindness, 85,* 3, 129-130.

Bernstein, G. B. (1979a). Integration of vision stimulation in the classroom I: Individual programming. *Education of the Visually Handicapped, 11,* 1, 14-18.

Bernstein, G. B. (1979b). Integration of vision stimulation in the classroom II: Group programming. *Education of the Visually Handicapped, 11,* 2, 39-48.

Bernstein, G. B. (1979c). Integration of vision stimulation in the classroom III: A total approach. *Education of the Visually Handicapped, 11, 3,* 80-85.

Bishop, V. E. (1986). *Selected anomalies and diseases of the eye.* Unpublished paper.

Bishop, V. E. (1988). Making choices in functional vision evaluations: "Noodles, needles, and haystacks." *Journal of Visual Impairment and Blindness, 82,* 3, 94-99.

Bongers, K. & Doudlah, A. (1972). Techniques for initiating visuomotor behavior in visually impaired retarded children. *Education of the Visually Handicapped, 4,* 3, 80-82.

Brilliant, R. (1983). Magnification in low vision aids made simple. *Journal of Visual Impairment and Blindness, 77,* 4, 169-171.

Browder, D. M. (1987). *Assessment of individuals with severe handicaps: An applied behavior approach to life skills assessment.* Baltimore: Paul Brooks.

Brown, C. J. & Langley, M. B. (1984). Diagnostic/prescriptive models for training inter-disciplinary personnel working with profoundly mentally handicapped learners. Talahassee, FL: Department of Education, Bureau of Education for Exceptional Students.

Burke, E. P. (1975.) *The assessment and training of visual behaviors in severely multihandicapped children.* Unpublished paper.

Burnette, J. (1987). *Adapting instructional materials for mainstreamed students: Issue brief 1.* Reston, VA: The Council for Exceptional Children, The ERIC/SEP Special Project on Interagency Information Dissemination.

Cassin, B. & Solomon, S. (1990). *Dictionary of eye terminology* (2nd ed.). Gainesville, FL: Triad.

Caton, H. (Ed.). (1991). *Print and braille literacy: Selecting appropriate learning media.* Louisville, KY: American Printing House for the Blind.

Chalkney, T. (1982). *Your eyes* (2nd ed.). Springfield, IL: Charles Thomas.

Chen, D., Friedman, C. T., & Calvello, G. (1990). *Parents and visually impaired infants (PAVII).* Louisville, KY: American Printing House for the Blind.

Cole, R. G. (1988). A unified approach to the optics of low vision aids-Part I. *Journal of Vision Rehabilitation, 2,* 1, 23-36.

Colenbrander, A. & Fletcher, D. C. (1990). Visual acuity measurement in low vision patients.*Journal of Vision Rehabilitation, 4,* 1, 1-9.

Connolly, M. B., Jan, J. E., & Cochran, D. (1991). Rapid recovery from cortical visual impairment following correction of prolonged shunt mulfunction in congenital hydrocephalus. *Archives of Neurology, 48,* 956-957.

Cook-Clampert, D. (1981). The development of self-concept in blind children. *Journal of Visual Impairment and Blindness, 75,* 6, 233-238.

Copeland, D., James, P., Richey, K., Seitz, W., & King, P. (1991). *Functional vision evaluation.* Mt. Pleasant, TX: Region VII Education Service Center.

Corn, A. L. (1980a). Functional environmental cues for the low vision individual. Excerpt from the *Interdisciplinary approach to low vision rehabilitation.* Prepared for the National Training Workshop in Low Vision, Chicago, August 25-27, 1980.

Corn, A. L. (1980b). Optical aids in the classroom. *Education of the Visually Handicapped, 12,* 4, 114-119.

Corn, A. L. (1983). Visual function: A theoretical model for individuals with low vision. *Journal of Visual Impairment and Blindness, 77,* 8, 373-377.

Corn, A. L. (1985). Strategies for the enhancement of visual functioning in individuals with fixed visual deficits: An interdisciplinary model. *Rehabilitation Literature, 46,* 1-2, 8-11.

References Continued

Corn, A. L. (1986). Low vision and visual efficiency. In G. T. Scholl (Ed.), *Foundations of education for blind and visually handicapped children and youth: Theory and practice.* New York: American Foundation for the Blind.

Corn, A. L. (1989a). Employing critical thinking strategies within a curriculum of critical things to think about for blind and visually impaired students. *Journal of Vision Rehabilitation, 3,* 4, 17-36.

Corn A. L. (1989b). Instruction in the use of vision for children and adults with low vision: A proposed program model. *RE:view, 21,* 1, 26-38.

Corn, A. L. (1986). Low vision and visual efficiency. In G. T. Scholl (Ed.), *Foundations of education for blind and visually handicapped children an youth: Theory and practice.* New York: American Foundation for the Blind.

Corn, A. L. & Bishop, V. E. (1991). Acquisition of practical knowledge by blind and visually impaired students in grades 8-12. *Journal of Visual Impairment and Blindness, 78,* 8, 352-355.

Corn, A. L. & Koenig, A. J. (1991). Least restrictive access to the visual environment. *Journal of Visual Impairment and Blindness, 85,* 195-197.

Corn, A. L. & Martinez, I. (n. d.). *When you have a visually handicapped child in your classroom: Suggestions for teachers.* New York: American Foundation for the Blind.

Corn, A. L. & Ryser, G. (1989). Access to print for students with low vision. *Journal of Visual Impairment and Blindness, 83,* 7, 340-349.

Coughlin, R. W. & Patz, A. (1978). Diabetic retinopathy: Nature and extent. *Journal of Visual Impairment and Blindness, 72,* 9, 343-347.

Cowan, C., & Sheplar, R. (1990). Teaching techniques for teaching young children to use low vision devices. *Journal of Visual Impairment and Blindness, 84,* 9, 419-421.

Cress, P. J., Spellman, C. R., DeBriere, T. J., Siemore, A. C., Northam, J. K., & Johnson, J. L. (1981). Vision screening for persons with severe handicaps, *TASH Journal, 6,* 41-50.

Davidson, I. F. & McKay, D. K. (1980). Using group procedures to develop social negotiation skills in blind young adults. *Journal of Visual Impairment and Blindness, 74 ,* 3, 97-101.

Davidson, I. F. & Simmons, J. N. (1984). Mediating the environment for young blind children: A conceptualization. *Journal of Visual Impairment and Blindness, 78,* 6, 251-255.

De Witt, J. C., Schreier, E. M., & Leventhal, J. D. (1988a). A look at closed circuit television systems (CCTV) for persons with low vision. *Journal of Visual Impairment and Blindness, 82,* 4, 151-160.

De Witt, J. C., Schreier, E. M., Leventhal, J. D., & Meyers, A. M. (1988b). A guide to selecting large print/enhanced image computer access hardware/software for persons with low vision. *Journal of Visual Impairment and Blindness, 82,* 10, 432-442.

Dickman, I. R. (1983). *Making life more livable: Simple adaptations for the homes of blind and visually impaired older adults.* New York: American Foundation for the Blind.

Directory of services for blind and visually impaired persons in the United States (23rd ed.). (1988). New York: American Foundation for the Blind.

Directory of living aids for the handicapped: A guide to products and devices for the handicapped. (1984). Santa Monica, CA: Ready Reference Press.

Dixon, H. A. (1989). He opened his eyes and smiled: A father's story of early intervention and stimulation. *Exceptional Parent,19,* 1, 18-23.

Donaldson, R. & Christiansen, J. (1990). Consultation and collaboration: A decision-making model. *Teaching Exceptional Children, 22,* 2, 22-25.

Downing, J. & Bailey, B. R. (1990a). Developing vision use within functional daily activities for students with visual and multiple disabilities. *RE:view, 21,* 4, 209-220.

Downing, J. & Bailey, B. R. (1990b). Sharing the responsibility: Using a transdisciplinary team approach to enhance the learning of students with severe disabilities. *Journal of Educational and Psychological Consultation, 1,* 3, 259-278.

Duncan, E., Prickett, H. T., Finkelstein, D., Vernon, M., & Hollingsworth, T. (1988). *Usher's syndrome: What it is, how to cope, and how to help.* Springfield, IL: Charles Thomas.

Eaglestein, A. & Rapaport, S. (1991). Prediction of low vision aid usage. *Journal of Visual Impairment and Blindness, 85,* 1, 31-33.

Educating students with visual impairments: Criteria for exemplary programs. (1991). Austin, TX: Texas Education Agency.

Efron, M. & DuBoff, B. R. (1975). *A vision guide for teachers of deaf-blind children.* Raleigh, NC: South Atlantic Regional Center for Services to Deaf-Blind Children.

References Continued

Efron, M., Miller-Wood, D. J., & Wood, T. A. (1989). Visual skill development for the functionally blind via closed circuit television. *Journal of Vision Rehabilitation, 3,* 4, 11-16.

Eldred, K. (1989). Use of a contact lens as a microscope. *Journal of Vision Rehabilitation, 3,* 2, 23-28.

Ellis, H. D., Young, A. W., & Markham, R. (1987). The ability of visually impaired children to read expressions and recognize faces. *Journal of Visual Impairment and Blindness, 81,* 10, 485-486.

Erhardt, R. P. (1990). *Developmental visual dysfunction: Models for assessment and management.* Tuscon, AR: Therapy Skill Builders.

Erin, J. N. (1986). Teachers of the visually handicapped: How can they best serve children with profound handicaps? *Education of the Visually Handicapped, 18,* 1, 15-25.

Erin, J. N. (1988). The teacher-consultant. *Education of the Visually Handicapped, 20,* 2, 57-64.

Erin, J. N. (1989). Cortical visual impairment: Implications for Service Delivery. *Journal of Vision Rehabilitation, 3,* 4, 1-10.

Erin, J. N., Dignan, K., & Brown, P. A. (1991). Are social skills teachable: A review of the literature. *Journal of Visual Impairment and Blindness, 85,* 2, 58-61.

Falvey, M. A. (1986). *Community-based curriculum: Instructional strategies for students with severe handicaps.* Baltimore: Paul Brooks.

Faubert, J., Overbury, O., Quillman, R. D., & Hill, P. (n. d.). *Spatial contrast sensitivity characteristics in the low vision population.* Unpublished paper.

Faye, E. E. (Ed.). (1984). *Clinical low vision* (2nd ed.). Boston: Little, Brown.

Fellows, R. R., Leguire, L. E., Rogers, G. L., & Bremer, D. L. (1986). A theoretical approach to vision stimulation. *Journal of Visual Impairment and Blindness, 80,* 8, 907-909.

Ferrell, K. A. (1984). A second look at sensory aids in early childhood. *Education of the Visually Handicapped, 16,* 3, 83-101.

Ferrell, K. A. (1985). *Reach out and teach.* New York: American Foundation for the Blind.

Ferrell, K. A. (1987). Step-by-step charts: Sequence of visual development. In L. Harrell & N. Akeson, *Preschool vision stimulation: It's more than a flashlight! Developmental perspectives for visually and multihandicapped infants and preschoolers.* New York: American Foundation for the Blind.

Fewell, R. R. (1983). Working with sensorially impaired children. In S. G. Garwood (Ed.), *Educating young handicapped children: A developmental approach* (2nd ed.). Rockville, MD: Aspen.

Ficocello, C. (1976). Vision stimulation for low functioning deaf-blind rubella children. *Teaching Exceptional Children, 8,* 3, 128-130.

Flodmark, O., Jan, J. E., Wong, P. K. H. (1990). Computed tomography of the brains of children with cortical visual impairment. *Development of Medicine and Child Neurology, 32,* 611-620.

Freed, B. (1990). Clinical categories of stand magnifiers: Measurement and application. *Journal of Vision Rehabilitation, 4,* 1, 49-52.

Freeman, R. D., Goetz, E., Richards, D. P., Groenveld, M., Blockberger, S., Jan, J. E., & Sykanda, A. M. (1989). Blind children's early emotional development: Do we know enough to help? *Child Care, Health and Development, 15,* 1, 3-28.

Friedman, C. T. (1989). Integrating infants. *Exceptional Parent, 19,* 1, 52-57.

Friedman, G. R. (1976). Distance low vision aids for primary school level children. *New Outlook for the Blind, 70,* 9, 376-379.

Functional vision evaluation for the academic student. (n. d.). Midland, TX: Region 18 Education Service Center.

Functional vision evaluation for the multihandicapped/non-academic/ nonverbal and/or 0-3 year old visually impaired child. (n. d.). Midland, TX: Region 18 Education Service Center.

Gardner, L. R. (1985). Low vision enhancement: The use of figure-ground reversals with visually impaired children. *Journal of Visual Impairment and Blindness, 79,* 2, 64-69.

Gardner, L. R. & Corn, A. (1984). Low vision: Topics of concern. In G. T. Scholl (Ed.), *Quality services for blind and visually handicapped learners: Statement of position.* Reston, VA: ERIC Clearinghouse on Handicapped and Gifted Children.

Gates, C. F. (1981). Vision assessment and stimulation for deaf-blind/ severely-profoundly handicapped children. *Viewpoints in Teaching and Learning, 57,* 1 43-53.

Genetic counselling. (1985). White Plains, NY: March of Dimes Birth Defects Foundation.

References Continued

Gittenger, J. & Asdourian, G. (1988). *Manual of clinical problems in ophthalmology with annotated key references.* Boston: Little, Brown.

Glanze, W. D., Anderson, K. N., & Anderson, L. E. (1987). *The Signet/ Mosby medical encyclopedia.* New York: C. V. Mosby

Goetz, L., & Gee, K. (1987a). Functional vision programming: A model for teaching visual behaviors in natural contexts. In L. Goetz, D. Guess, & K. Stremel-Campbell (Eds.), *Innovative program design for individuals with dual sensory impairments.* Baltimore: Paul Brooks.

Goetz, L., & Gee, K. (1987b). Teaching visual attention in functional contexts: Acquisition and generalization of complex visual motor skills. *Journal of Visual Impairment and Blindness, 81,* 3, 115-117.

Goodrich, G. L. & Jose, R. T. (1990). *Low vision - the reference: A literature database.* Tulsa, OK: The Low Vision Center.

Graves, W., Maxson, J., & McCaa, C. (1988). Assessing the environment of low vision persons: A validation of procedure. *Journal of Visual Impairment and Blindness, 82,* 9, 361-365.

Greenblatt, S. L. (1989). *Providing services for people with vision loss: A multidisciplinary perspective.* Lexington, MA: Resources for Rehabilitation.

Greig, D. E., West, M. L., & Overby, O. (1986). Successful use of low vision aids: Visual and psychological factors. *Journal of Visual Impairment and Blindness, 80,* 10, 985-988.

Gregory, R. L. (1972). *Eye and brain: The psychology of seeing.* New York: McGraw-Hill.

Griffin-Shirley, N., McNeely, E., & Karwisch, A. (1990). Videotape simulations to teach staff of long-term care facilities about residents' vision loss. *Journal of Visual Impairment and Blindness, 84,* 10, 530-531.

Groenveld, M., Jan, J. E., & Leader, P. (1990). Observations on the habilitation of children with cortical visual impairment. *Journal of Visual Impairment and Blindness, 84,* 1, 11-15.

Haith, M. M. (1990). Progress in understanding of sensory and perceptual processes in early infancy. *Merrill-Palmer Quarterly, 36,* 1, 1-26.

Hall, A. P. & Bailey, I. L. (1989). A model for training vision functioning. *Journal of Visual Impairment and Blindness, 83,* 8, 390-396.

Hall, A. P., Kekelis, L. S., & Bailey, I. L. (1986). *Development of an assessment program and intervention guidelines for visually impaired children.* Berkeley, CA: Center for the Study of Visual Impairment, School of Optometry, University of California.

Hall, A. P., Orel-Bixler, D., & Haegerstrom-Portnoy, G. (1991). Special visual assessment techniques for multiply handicapped persons. *Journal of Visual Impairment and Blindness, 85,* 1, 23-29.

Harley, R. K., Garcia, M., Williams, M. F. (1989). The educational placement of visually impaired children. *Journal of Visual Impairment and Blindness, 83,* 10, 512-516.

Harley R. K. & Lawrence, G. A. (1977). *Visual impairments in the schools.* Springfield, IL: Charles Thomas.

Harley, R. K., Truan, M. B., & Sanford, Z. D. (1987). *Communication skills for visually impaired learners.* Springfield, IL: Charles Thomas.

Harrell, L. & Akeson, N. (1987). *Preschool vision stimulation: It's more than a flashlight!* New York: American Foundation for the Blind.

Hazekamp, J. & Huebner, K. M. (Eds.). (1989). *Program planning and evaluation for blind and visually impaired students: National guidelines for educational excellence.* New York: American Foundation for the Blind.

Heitzmann, C. A. & Ward, R. (1990). Vision rehabilitation with cognitively impaired patients. *Journal of Vision Rehabilitation, 4,* 1, 11-18.

Hoben, M. & Lindstrom V. (1980). Evidence of isolation in the mainstream. *Journal of Visual Impairment and Blindness, 74,* 8, 289-292.

Hofstetter, H. W. (1991). Efficacy of low vision services for visually impaired children. *Journal of Visual Impairment and Blindness, 85,* 1, 20-22.

Horner, R. H., Meyer, L. H., & Fredricks, H. D. (1986). *Education of learners with severe handicaps: Exemplary service strategies.* Baltimore: Paul Brooks.

Hoyt, S. H. (1978). Rehabilitation teachers can form a simplified delivery system for low vision aids. *Journal of Visual Impairment and Blindness, 72,* 8, 322-324.

Hupp, S. C. & Rosen, S. (1985). The team approach to designing instruction for visually impaired multiply handicapped children: A decision-making paradigm. *Education of the Visually Handicapped, 17,* 3, 85-96.

Jackson, R. M. (1983a). Early educational use of optical aids: A cautionary note. *Education of the Visually Handicapped, 15,* 1, 20-29.

Jackson, R. M. (1983b). The importance of perceptual activity in the development of visually handicapped infants and preschoolers. In M. E. Mulholland & M. V. Wuster (Eds.), *"Help me to become everything that I can be." Proceedings from the North American conference on visually handicapped infants and preschool children.* New York: American Foundation for the Blind.

Jacobs, R. (1990). Screen color and reading performance on closed-circuit television. *Journal of Visual Impairment and Blindness, 84,* 10, 569-572.

Jampolsky, A., Brabyn, J., Lewis, A., & Winderl, M. (1989). Two experimental low vision illumination aids. *Journal of Vision Rehabilitation, 3,* 3, 33-37.

Jan, J. E., Freeman, R. D., & Scott, E. P. (1977). *Visual impairments in children and adolescents.* New York: Grune and Stratton.

Jan. J. E., Groenveld, M., & Sykanda, A. M. (1990). Light-gazing by visually impaired children. *Developmental Medicine and Child Neurology, 32,* 755-759.

Jan, J. E., Groenveld, M., Sykanda, A. M., & Hoyt, C. S. (1987). Behavioral characteristics of children with permanent cortical visual impairment. *Developmental Medicine and Child Neurology, 29,* 571-576.

Jan, J. E., Wong, P. K. H., Groenveld, M., Flodmark, O., & Hoyt, C. S. (1986). Travel vision: "Collicular visual ystem?". *Pediatric Neurology, 2,* 359-362.

Jose, R. T. (Ed.). (1983). *Understanding low vision.* New York: American Foundation for the Blind.

Jose, R. T. & Bauman, N. (n. d.). *Overview of ocular diseases and disorders.* Unpublished Paper.

Jose, R. T., Labossiere, S., & Small, M. (1987). Project D.O.V.E.S.: Delivering optimum vision and education services. *Journal of Vision Rehabilitation, 1,* 1, 5-21.

Jose, R. T., Smith, A. J., & Shane, K. G. (1980) Evaluating and stimulating vision in the multiply impaired. *Journal of Visual Impairment and Blindness, 74,* 1, 2-8.

Jose, R. T., Spitzberg, L. A., & Kuether, C. L. (1989). A behind the lens reversed (BTLR) telescope. *Journal of Vision Rehabilitation, 3,* 2, 37-46.

Kalloniatis, M. & Johnston, A. W. (1990a). Color vision characteristics of low vision children. *Optometry & Vision Science, 67,* 3, 166-168.

Kalloniatis, M. & Johnston, A. W. (1990b). Visual characteristics of low vision children. *Optometry & Vision Science, 67,* 1, 38-48.

Kastner, B. D. (1990). Rehabilitative management of maculopathies. *Journal of Vision Rehabilitation, 3,* 4, 33-47.

Kelleher, D. K. (1979). Orientation to low vision aids. *Journal of Visual Impairment and Blindness, 73,* 5, 161-166.

Kelly, P. T. (1977). *Dealing with dilemma: A manual for genetic counselors.* New York: Springer-Verlag.

Kiester, E. (1990). *AIDS and vision loss.* New York: American Foundation for the Blind.

Knowlton, M. (1986). Ultraviolet light: Some considerations for vision stimulation. *Education of the Visually Handicapped, 17,* 4, 147-153.

Knowlton, M. (1987). Assessing contrast: Quantifying the environment. *Journal of Vision Rehabilitation, 1,* 2, 9-13.

Knowlton, M. & Normandin, J. (1987). A method for assessing acuity in the natural environment. *Journal of Visual Impairment and Blindness, 81,* 9, 435-436.

Knowlton, M., Sorensen, M., & Grafsgaard, C. (1987). *Improving services for handicapped children through networking.* Symposium conducted at the Annual Meeting of the Council for Exceptional Children, Chicago.

Knowlton, M. & Woo, I. (1989a). Assessment of functional color perception. *Journal of Vision Rehabilitation, 3,* 2, 5-22.

Knowlton, M. & Woo, I. (1989b). Functional color vision deficits and performance of children on an educational task. *Education of the Visually Handicapped, 20,* 4, 156-162.

Koenig, A. J. & Holbrook, M. C. (1989). Determining the reading medium for students with visual impairments: A diagnostic teaching approach. *Journal of Visual Impairment and Blindness, 83,* 6, 296-302.

Koenig, A. J. & Holbrook, M. C. (1991). Determining the reading medium for visually impaired students via diagnostic teaching. *Journal of Visual Impairment and Blindness, 85,* 2, 61-68.

Koenig, A. J. & Rex, E. J. (1983). Assessment of optacon reading: A preliminary investigation. *Journal of Visual Impairment and Blindness, 77,* 2, 56-60.

References Continued

Koenig, A. J. & Ross, D. B. (1991). A procedure to evaluate the relative effectiveness of reading in large and regular print. *Journal of Visual Impairment and Blindess, 84,* 5, 198-204.

Kunz, J. R. M. (Ed.). (1982). *The American Medical Association family medical guide.* New York: Random House.

Lagrow, S. J. & Matson, J. L. (1984). Increasing recognition distance and assessing generalized effects in visually impaired persons. *Journal of Visual Impairment and Blindness, 78,* 6, 256-260.

Lang, M. A. & Sullivan, C. (1986). Adapting home environments for visually impaired and blind children. *Children's Environments Quarterly, 3,* 11, 50-54.

Langley, M. B. (1980). *Functional vision inventory for the multiply and severely handicapped.* Chicago: Stoelting.

Langley, M. B. (in press). *Potential assessment of visual efficiency* (working title). Louisville, KY: American Printing House for the Blind.

Langley, M. B. & DuBose, R. F. (1976). Functional vision screening for severely handicapped children. *The New Outlook for the Blind, 70,* 8, 346-350.

Legge, G. E., Rubin, G. S., Pelli, D. G., Schleske, M. M., Luebker, A., & Ross, J. A. (1988). Understanding low vision reading. *Journal of Visual Impairment and Blindness, 82,* 2, 54-59.

Levack, N. (Ed.). (in press). *Basic skills for community living: A curriculum for students with visual impairments and multiple disabilities.* Austin, TX: Texas School for the Blind and Visually Impaired.

Levner, H. (1985). *I keep five pairs of glasses in a flower pot.* Roslyn, NY: National Association for the Visually Handicapped.

Lippmann, O., Corn, A. L., & Lewis, M. C. (1988). Bioptic telescopic spectacles and driving performance: A study in Texas. *Journal of Visual Impairment and Blindness, 82,* 5, 182-187.

Lighthouse low vision catalog: Optical devices, products, services (6th ed.). (1988). Long Island City, NY: The Lighthouse.

Living with low vision: A resource guide for people with sight loss. (1990). Lexington, MA: Resources for Rehabilitation.

Lloyd, J. H. (1984). Use of telescopic aids for vocational purposes. *Journal of Visual Impairment and Blindness, 78,* 5, 216-220.

Loumiet, R. & Levack, N. (1991). *Independent living: A curriculum with adaptations for students with visual impairments.* Austin, TX: Texas School for the Blind and Visually Impaired.

Lowenfeld, B. (1981). *Berthold Lowenfeld on blindness and blind people: Selected papers.* New York: American Foundation for the Blind.

Low vision question and answers: Definitions, devices, and services. (1987). New York: American Foundation for the Blind.

Lundervold, D., Levin, L. M., & Irvin, L. K. (1987). Rehabilitation of visual impairments: A critical review. *Clinical Psychology Review, 7,* 169-185.

Mangold, S. S. (Ed.). (1982). *A teacher's guide to the special educational needs of blind and visually handicapped children.* New York: American Foundation for the Blind.

Mangold, S. S. (1988). Nurturing high self-esteem in adolescents with visual handicaps. *Journal of Vision Rehabilitation, 2,* 3, 5-9.

Mangold, S. S. & Mangold, P. N. (1983). The adolescent visually impaired female. *Journal of Visual Impairment and Blindness, 77,* 6, 250-255.

Mangold, S. S. & Mangold, P. N. (1989). Selecting the most appropriate primary learning medium for students with functional vision. *Journal of Visual Impairment and Blindness, 83,* 6, 294-296.

Maplesden, C. (1984). A subjective approach to eccentric viewing training. *Journal of Visual Impairment and Blindness, 78,* 1, 5-6.

Martin, S. F. (1990). Optometric vision therapy for low vision patients. *Journal of Vision Rehabilitation, 4,* 1, 53-57.

McAllister, B. (1990). A model for the visual evaluation of partially sighted preschoolers. *Journal of Vision Rehabilitation, 4,* 4, 5-10.

Mellor, C. M. (1981). *Aids for the 80s: What they are and what they do.* New York: American Foundation for the Blind.

Mercer, D. (1991a). *So what does this kid see? Performing and reporting functional vision assessments.* Unpublished paper.

Mercer, D. (1991b). *So you've got a visually handicapped kid in your classroom.* Unpublished paper.

Mettler, R. (1990). An integrated, problem-solving approach to low vision training. *Journal of Visual Impairment and Blindness, 84,* 4, 171-177.

Myers, P. I. & Hammill, D. D. (1990). *Learning disabilities: Basic concepts, assessment practice, and instructional strategies* (4th ed.). Austin, TX: Pro•Ed.

Michael, M. G. & Paul, P. V. (1991). Early intervention for infants with deaf-blindness. *Exceptional Children, 1,* 200-209.

Miller-Wood, D., Efron, M., & Wood, T. (1990). Use of closed-circuit television with a severely visually impaired young child. *Journal of Visual Impairment and Blindness, 84,* 10, 559-565.

Moore, S. (1984). The need for programs and services for visually handicapped infants. *Education for the Visually Handicapped, 15,* 2, 48-55.

Morse, M. T. (1990). Cortical visual impairment in young children with multiple disabilities. *Journal of Visual Impairment and Blindness, 84,* 5, 200-203.

Morse, M. T. (1991). Visual gaze behaviors: Considerations in working with visually impaired multiply handicapped children. *RE:view, 13,* 1, 5-15.

Morris, O. F. (1981). Teacher assessment of visual functioning. *Education of the Visually Handicapped, 13,* 2, 42-50.

Morrisette, D., Goodrich, D., & Marmor, M. (1985). A study of the effectiveness of the wide angle mobility light. *Journal of Visual Impairment and Blindness, 79,* 3, 109-111.

Mosler, V. I. (1986). Night vision aid option: Streamlights. *Journal of Visual Impairment and Blindness, 80,* 10, 1005-1006.

Muranaka, Y., Furuta, N., Aoki, S., & Gohke, K. (1985). Use of the simplified color video magnifier by young children with severely impaired vision. *Journal of Visual Impairment and Blindness, 79,* 9, 319-395.

Myers, P. I. & Hammill, D. D. (1990). *Learning disabilities: Basic concepts, assessment practices, and instructional strategies* (4th ed.). Austin, TX: Pro•Ed.

Myers, W. A. (1971). Color discriminability for partially seeing children. *Exceptional Children, 37,* 223-228.

Needham, W. E. (1988). Cognitive distortions in acquired visual loss. *Journal of Vision Rehabilitation, 2,* 3, 45-523.

Needham, W. E. & Ehmer, M. N. (1980). Irrational thinking and adjustment to loss of vision. *Journal of Visual Impairment and Blindness, 74,* 2, 57-61.

Nelson, D. (1984). *Children with autism and other pervasive disorders of development and behavior.* Thorofare, NJ: Charles B. Slack.

Nemshick, L. A., Vernon, M. C., & Ludman, F. (1986). The impact of retinitis pigmentosa on young adults: Psychological, educational, vocational and social considerations. *Journal of Visual Impairment and Blindness, 80,* 7, 859-862.

Newcomer, P. & Hammill, D. (1973). Visual perception of motor impaired children: Implications for assessment. *Exceptional Children, 39,* 4, 335-338.

O'Dea, A. F. & Mayhall, C. A. (1988). Delayed manifestations of congenital rubella. *Journal of Visual Impairment and Blindness, 82,* 9, 379-381.

Orel-Bixler, D., Haegerstrom-Portnoy, G., & Hall, A. (1989). Visual assessment of the multiply handicapped patient. *Optometry &Vision Science, 66,* 8, 530-536.

Orelove, F. P. & Sobesy, D. (1987). *Educating children with multiple disabilities: A transdisciplinary approach.* Baltimore: Paul Brooks.

Overby, O., Goodrich, G. L. Quillman, R. D., & Faubert, J. (1989). Perceptual assessment in low vision: Evidence for a hierarchy of skills? *Journal of Visual Impairment and Blindness, 83,* 2, 109-113.

Parsons, S. (1987). Locus of control and adaptive behavior in visually impaired children. *Journal of Visual Impairment and Blindness, 81,* 9, 429-432.

Pavan-Langston, D. (1985.) *Manual of ocular diagnosis and therapy* (2nd ed.). Boston: Little, Brown.

Peli, E., Arend, L. E., & Timberlake, G. T. (1986). Computerized image enhancement for visually impaired persons: New technology, new possibilities. *Journal of Visual Impairment and Blindness, 80,* 7, 849-854.

Perle, T. (1976). A matter of adjustment: A personal reaction to visual loss. *Journal of Visual Impairment and Blindness, 70,* 7, 255-258.

Porter, F. I., Demer, J. L., Goldberg, J., Jenkins, H. A., & Schmidt, K. (1987). Developing a methodology for predicting successful visual rehabilitation with spectacle magnifiers. *Journal of Visual Rehabilitation, 1,* 1, 22-35.

Potenski, D. (1983). Use of black light in training retarded, multiply handicapped, deaf-blind children. *Journal of Visual Impairment and Blindness, 77,* 7, 347-348.

Programs for guidelines for visually impaired individuals (rev. ed.). (1987). Sacramento, CA: California State Department of Education.

Prokopich, L. (1989). Visual rehabilitation in homonymous hemianopia due to cerebral vascular accident. *Journal of Vision Rehabilitation, 3,* 2, 29-35.

Raver-Lampman, S. A. (1990). Effect of gaze direction on evaluation of visually impaired children by informed respondents. *Journal of Visual Impairment and Blindness, 84,* 2, 67-70.

Read, L. F. (1989). An examination of social skills of blind kindergarten children. *Education of the Visually Handicapped, 20,* 4, 142-155.

Rehabilitation resource manual: Vision. (1990). Lexington, MA: Resources for Rehabilitation.

Resource manual for functional vision evaluation. (1984). Austin, TX: Texas Education Agency.

Rex, E. J. (1989). Issues related to literacy of legally blind learners. *Journal of Visual Impairment and Blindness, 83,* 6, 306-313.

Riccardi, V. M. (1978). *The genetic approach to human disease.* New York: Oxford University Press.

Rickelman, R. N. & Blaylock, J. N. (1983). *Journal of Visual Impairment and Blindness, 77,* 1, 8-11.

Robertson, R., Jan. J. E., & Wong, P. K. H. (1986). Electroencephalograms of children with permanent cortical visual impairment. *The Canadian Journal of Neurological Science, 13,* 256-261.

Robinson, G. A. (1985). Best practices in assessment of visually handicapped students. In A. Thomas & J. Grimes (Eds.), *Best practices in school psychology.* Kent, OH: National Association of School Psychologists.

Rogow, S. M. (1988). *Helping the visually impaired child with developmental problems: Effective practice in home, school, and community.* New York: Teacher's College Press.

Rogow, S. M. & Rathwell, D. (1989). Seeing and knowing: An investigation of visual perception among children with severe visual impairments. *Journal of Vision Rehabilitation, 3,* 3, 55-66.

Rosner, J. (1988). Parents as screeners for strabismus in their children. *Journal of Visual Impairment and Blindness, 82,* 5, 193-196.

Sacks, S. Z. & Gaylord-Ross, R. (1989). Peer-mediated and teacher directed social skills training for visually impaired students. *Behavior Therapy, 20,* 619-638.

Sacks, S. Z. & Reardon, M. P. (1989). Maximizing social integration for students with visual handicaps. In R. Gaylord-Ross (Ed.), *Integration strategies for students with handicaps.* Baltimore: Paul Brooks.

Saez, P. E. (1989). Integration of blind and visually impaired children: The philosophy. *Journal of Visual Impairment and Blindness, 83,* 1, 54-56.

Sailor, W., Utley, B., Goetz, L., Gee, K. J., Baldwin, M., Hatlen, P., & Peterson, J. (1980). *Vison assessment and program manual.* San Francisco: Bay Area Severely Handicapped Deaf Blind Project, San Francisco State University.

Scholl, G. T. (Ed.). (1986). *Foundations of education for blind and visually handicapped children and youth: Theory and practice.* New York: American Foundation for the Blind.

Scholl, G. T. & Weihl, C. A. (1979). A survey of special curricular areas to be included in day programs for visually handicapped pupils. *Education of the Visually Handicapped, 11,* 1, 18-23.

Schroeder, F. (1989). Literacy: The key to opportunity. *Journal of Visual Impairment and Blindness, 83,* 6, 290-293.

Scott, R. A. (1969). The socialization of blind children. In D. Goslin (Ed.), *Handbook of socialization theory and research.* Chicago: Rand McNally.

Shindell, S., (1988). Low vision: a social disease. *Journal of Vision Rehabilitation, 2,* 3, 77-85.

Shull, L. E. & Kuyk, T. (1990). Wide angle mobility light (WAML) follow up. *Journal of Visual Impairment and Blindness, 84,* 2, 78-79.

Sicurella, V. J. (1977). Color contrast as an aid for visually impaired persons. *Journal of Visual Impairment and Blindness, 71,* 6, 252-257.

Silberman, R. K. (1981). Assessment and evaluation of visually handicapped students. *Journal of Visual Impairment and Blindness, 75,* 3, 109-114.

Silberman, R. K. & Sowell, V. (1987). The visually impaired student with learning disabilities: Strategies for success in language arts. *Education of the Visually Handicapped, 18,* 4, 139-150.

Simmons, J. N. & Davidson, I. F. (1984). Mediation for young blind children: An introduction to the literature. *Journal of Visual Impairment and Blindness, 78,* 3, 118-120.

Singh, T. B. (1984). A study of the locus of control of visually handicapped persons. *Psychological Studies, 29,* 1, 93-95.

Siperstein, G. N. & Bak, J. J. (1980). Improving children's attitudes toward blind peers. *Journal of Visual Impairment and Blindness, 74,* 4, 132-134.

Smith, A. J. & Cote, K. S. (1982). *Look at me: A resource manual for the development of residual vision in multiply impaired children.* Philadelphia: Pennsylvania College of Optometry Press.

Spitzberg, L. A., Jose, R. T., & . Kuether, C. L. (1989). A new ergonomically designed prism stand magnifier. *Journal of Vision Rehabilitation, 3,* 4, 47-51.

Spitzberg, L. A., Kuether, C. L., & Jose, R. T. (1987). The new writing magnifier. *Journal of Vision Rehabilitation, 1,* 2, 23-27.

Spungin, S. J. (1989). *Braille literacy: Issues for blind persons, families, professionals, and producers of braille.* New York: American Foundation for the Blind.

Stein, H. A., Slatt, B. J., & Cook, P. (1982). *Manual of ophthalmic terminology.* St. Louis: C. V. Mosby.

Stein, H. A., Slatt, B. J., & Stein R. M. (1987). *Ophthalmo terminology: Speller and vocabulary builder* (2nd ed.). St. Louis: C. V. Mosby.

Stephens, O. (1989). Braille - implications for living. *Journal of Visual Impairment and Blindness, 83,* 6, 288-289.

Stratton, J. M. (1990). The principle of least-restrictive materials. *Journal of Visual Impairment and Blindness, 84,* 1, 3-5.

Suttie, A. J., & Greenhalgh, R. (1985). A method of assessing visually impaired person's ability to use a closed circuit television reading machine. *Journal of Visual Impairment and Blindness, 79,* 8, 347-353.

Swallow, R. (1976). *The low vision child in the classroom.* Unpublished paper.

Swallow, R., Mangold, S, & Mangold, P. (Eds.). (1978). *AFB practice report: Informal assessment of developmental skills for visually handicapped students.* New York: American Foundation for the Blind.

Swallow, R., Spungin, S., & Chase, J. (1977). *AFB practice report: Collection of three papers.* New York: American Foundation for the Blind.

Swenson, A. M. (1988). Using an integrated literacy curriculum with beginning braille readers. *Journal of Visual Impairment and Blindness, 83,* 7, 366-383.

Sykes, K. S. (1971). A comparison of the effectiveness of standard print in facilitating the reading of visually impaired students. *Education of the Visually Handicapped, 3,* 4, 97-106.

Szlyk, J. P., Arditi, A., Coffey Bucci, P., & Laderman, D. (1990). Self-report in functional assessment of low vision. *Journal of Visual Impairment and Blindness, 84,* 2, 61-66.

Tait, P. E. (1989). Optic nerve hypoplasia: A review of the literature. *Journal of Visual Impairment and Blindness, 83,* 4, 207-211.

Tapp, K. L., Wilhelm, J. G., & Loveless, L. J. (1991). *A guide to curriculum planning for visually impaired students.* Madison, WI: Wisconson Department of Public Instruction.

Taylor, E. J., Anderson, D. M., Patwell, J. M., Plaut, K., & McCullough, K. (Eds.). (1988). *Dorland's illustrated medical dictionary* (27th ed.). Philadelphia: W. B. Saunders.

Turner, B. & Erchul W. (1987). Visually impaired children: Psychoeducational assessment issues. *School Psychology International, 8,* 2-3, 105-115.

Tuttle, D. W. (1984). *Self-esteem and adjusting with blindness: The process of responding to life's demands.* Springfield, IL: Charles Thomas.

Tuttle, D. W. (1986). Educational Programming. In G. T. School (Ed.), *Foundations of education for blind and visually handicapped children and youth: Theory and practice.* New York: American Foundation for the Blind.

Trief, E., Duckman, R., Morse, A. R., & Silberman, R. K. (1989). Retinopathy of prematurity. *Journal of Visual Impairment and Blindness, 83,* 10, 500-504.

Understanding eye language. (1977). New York: National Society for the Prevention of Blindness.

Upsal Low Vision Team. (n. d.). *Functional implications of diseases.* Unpublished paper.

Utley, B. N., Duncan, D., Strain, P., & Scanlon, K. (1983). Effects of contingent and noncontingent vision stimulation on visual fixation in multiply handicapped children. *TASH Journal,* 8, 29-42.

Utley, B. N. & Ferrell, K. A. (1989). *An assessment and intervention model to promote the integrated use of vision and visual motor skills.* Unpublished paper.

Vaughan, D. & Ashbury, T. (1980). *General ophthalmology* (9th ed.) Los Altos, CA: Lang Medical.

Vernon, M. (n. d.). *Answers to your questions about Usher's syndrome.* Baltimore: National Retinitis Pigmentosa Foundation.

Visual aids and informational material (8th ed.). (1991). New York: National Association for the Visually Handicapped.

Ward, M. E. (1986). Planning the individualized educational program. In G. T. Scholl (Ed.), *Foundations of education for blind and visually handicapped children and youth: Theory and practice.* New York: American Foundation for the Blind.

Warren, D. H. (1984). *Blindness and early childhood development.* (2nd ed. rev.). New York: American Foundation for the Blind.

Watson, G. (1989). Competencies and a bibliography addressing students' use of low vision devices. *Journal of Visual Impairment and Blindness, 83,* 3, 160-163.

Watson, G., Baldasare, J., & Whittaker, S. (1990). The validity and clinical uses of the Pepper visual skills reading test. *Journal of Visual Impairment and Blindness, 84,* 3, 119-124.

Whiting, S., Jan, J. E., Wong, P. K. H., Flodmark, O., Ferrell, K., & McCormick, A. Q. (1985). Permanent cortical visual impairment in children. *Developmental Medicine and Child Neurology, 27,* 730-739.

Wiener, W. & Vopata, A. (1980). Suggested curriculum for distance vision training with optical aids. *Journal of Visual Impairment and Blindness, 74,* 2, 49-56.

Yarkovishin, V. M. (1988). Coping with macular degeneration: From an optical perspective. *Journal of Visual Impairment and Blindness, 82,* 4, 127-128.

Yeadon, A. (Ed.). (1988). *International low vision directory.* Philadelphia: Institute for the Visually Impaired, Pennsylvania College of Optometry.

Yeadon, A. & Grayson, D. (1979). *Living with impaired vision: An introduction.* New York: American Foundation for the Blind.

Zahn, J. (1987). Usher's syndrome: Psychological and electrodiagnostic data on three families. *Journal of Visual Rehabilitation, 1,* 2, 15-21.

Zahn, J. (1989). Age-related maculopathy (ARM): The rehabilitation process. *Journal of Visual Rehabilitation, 3,* 1, 25-33.

Zambone, A. (1989). Serving the young child with visual impairments: An overview of disability impact and intervention needs. *Infants and Young Children, 2,* 2, 11-23.

Zimmerman, D. R. (1977). Birth defects and visual impairment. *Journal of Visual Impairment and Blindness, 71,* 1, 2-11.

mental retardation   139
microcephaly   116, 117, 119, 148, 238
microphthalmia, microphthalmos   116, 117, 119,
    120, **137**
microscopes 83
minus lens   30
mobility   238
Möbius' syndrome   119
monochromacy   144
monocular   80-81, 238
motor behaviors   242
Motor-Free Visual Perception Test (MVPT)   232
mouthing   179
movement disorders   162-163, 170
multisensory approach   100, 238
muscle imbalance   132, 146
muscle weakness   132, 155, 170, 171
myasthemia gravis   141
myopia   115-117, 119, **138**, 142, 143

N

near point of convergence   29, 238
near senses   172
near vision   29, 41, 42, 238
nearsightedness   138
neurofibromatosis   115, 148
neurological   238
neuromuscular   238
neuronal ceroid-lipofuscinosis   116
night blindness   116, 118, 142
night-vision scope   85
non-optical devices   86
Norrie's disease   115, 119
null point   238
nystagmus   26, 27, 117, 120, 121, 124, 127, 129,
    131, 136, 138, 139, 144, 147, 186

O

ocular fixation   168
ocular-motor control   155, 166, 168
oculocerebrorenal   118
oculogram   26
Ocutricin   149
olfaction   172
opacities   125, 130
ophthalmologist   23, 34, 238
optic atrophy   115-117, 136, 139, 140, 148
optic disc   105, 107, 126, 139, 140
optic nerve   26, 39, 105-107, 124, 129, 139
optic atrophy   120, 136, 139
optic hydroplasia   117, 119, 122, 131, 139
optical abilities   106, 110
optical character recognition systems (scanners)   89

optical devices   34, 47, 79, 199
optical righting reactions   167
optician   238
optokinetic drum   27, 32, 232
optometrist   23, 34, 37, 239
orientation & mobility   239

P

papilledemia   **140**, 148
partial participation   59, 239
Patau's syndrome   115, 119
Pediatric Low Vision Test Chart   229
perception   52, 175, 239
peripheral vision   31, 122, 136, 137, 142, 144, 239
Peter's anomaly   119
photocopy enlarging   91
photography   91
photophobia   116, 118, 121, 124, 125, 127-130,
    137, 142, 144, 145, 147, **239**
photoreceptors   105, 107
phthisis bulbi   140
physical feedback   199
Pilocarpine   149
PL (Public Law)   27
plus lens   28, 30
POHS (Presumed Ocular Histoplasmosis Syndrom)
    134
poor balance   155, 166, 170
poor posture   156, 170
position in space   155, 192
posterior   239
posterior chamber   106, 107
postural control   166-171
posture   156, 164
preferential looking   27, 32
presbyopia   140
prescription lenses   24, 28
presumed ocular histoplasmosis syndrome   134
print   47, 77
prism diopter   28, 29
prism   239
Program to Develop Efficiency in
    Visual Functioning   64
programming   4-17, 238
    challenge   6
    cortical visual impairments   16-17
    different student groups   11
    educational   8
    students who are near, at, or above their
        developmental level   12
    students who are significantly
        developmentally delayed   14
projectors   91

vitreous   106, 107, 132
von Recklinghausen's disease   148

W

WAML (Wide Angle Mobility Light)   91
Wells Standard Test Types Cards 230
Wilm's Tumor   125, **147**

X

X-linked   118, 119, 122, 124, 127, 129, 144, 242

Z

Zellweger's syndrome   122